Fibromyalgia:

A COMPREHENSIVE APPROACH

Fibromyalgia:

A COMPREHENSIVE APPROACH

What You Can Do About Chronic Pain and Fatigue

Miryam Ehrlich Williamson

FOREWORD BY DAVID A. NYE, M.D.

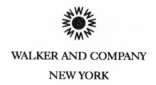

WALKER AND COMPANY

NEW YORK

In memory of my father,

HERMAN TRAMER EHRLICH (1904–1961),

whose face but never his words told of his pain.

First published in the United States of America in 1996
by Walker Publishing Company, Inc.

Published simultaneously in Canada
by Thomas Allen & Son Canada, Limited, Markham, Ontario

Library of Congress Cataloging-in-Publication Data
Williamson, Miryam Ehrlich.
Fibromyalgia: a comprehensive approach: what you can do about chronic pain and fatigue/Miryam Ehrlich Williamson; foreword by David A. Nye.
p. cm.
Includes index.
ISBN 0-8027-7484-9 (pbk.)
1. Fibromyalgia—Popular works. I. Title.
RC927.3.W53 1996
616.7′4—dc20 96-3251
CIP

Book design by M. J. DiMassi

Printed in the United States of America

18 20 19

CONTENTS

FOREWORD

Fibromyalgia is a common and disabling disorder affecting 2 to 4 percent of the population, women more often than men. Despite the condition's frequency, the diagnosis is often missed. Patients with fibromyalgia usually ache all over, sleep poorly, are stiff on waking, and are tired all day. They are prone to headaches, memory and concentration problems, dizziness, numbness and tingling, itching, fluid retention, crampy abdominal or pelvic pain, diarrhea, and several other symptoms.

There are no diagnostic lab or X-ray abnormalities, but a physician can confirm the diagnosis by finding multiple tender points in characteristic locations. Fibromyalgia often runs in families, suggesting an inherited predisposition. It may lie dormant until triggered by an injury, stress, or sleep disturbance.

Fibromyalgia has mistakenly been thought to be either an inflammatory or a psychiatric condition. However, no evidence of inflammation or arthritis has been found, and it is now believed that depression and anxiety, when present, are more often the result than the cause of fibromyalgia.

There is better evidence that fibromyalgia is due to an abnormality of deep sleep. Abnormal brain waves in deep sleep have been found in many patients with fibromyalgia. Fibromyalgia-like symptoms can be produced in normal volunteers by depriving them of deep sleep for a few days. Growth hormone, important in maintaining good muscle and other soft tissue health, tends to be low in patients with fibromyalgia. This hormone is produced almost exclusively in deep sleep, and its production is increased by exercise.

I should point out though that although this is my favorite among the theories of the cause of fibromyalgia, there are several other viable ones, and there is probably not a majority of fibromyalgia researchers that support any one theory.

Taking medication by itself has relatively little effect on fibromyalgia symptoms. Successful treatment requires active involvement of the patient in his or her care, including:

- Medication to improve deep sleep
- Regular sleep hours and an adequate amount of sleep
- Daily gentle aerobic exercise
- Avoidance of undue physical and emotional stress
- Treatment of any coexisting sleep disorders
- Patient education

If any of these steps is omitted, the chance of significant improvement is greatly reduced.

It often takes a lot of fiddling with the dose to get it exactly right, and frequently it will be necessary to try several medications in succession or sometimes in combination. The medication may eventually become less effective and the dose may then need to be increased slightly. Most patients will need to continue on medication indefinitely.

There are several herbal and other alternative remedies that some patients feel are helpful. I can't recommend them simply because they haven't been adequately studied for efficacy or long-term harm, but I don't discourage patients from using them if they find them helpful.

Patients who learn as much as possible about this disorder usually do better than those who don't. Fibromyalgia sufferers often elicit less sympathy and support than they deserve from family, friends, and employers because of the lack of outward evidence of disease. Many have been told by physicians that there is nothing wrong with them or that it is "all in your head," which can be demoralizing. For these reasons, and just because it is good to know that you are not alone, attending a support group can be valuable. Your physician or local hospital may be able to direct you to a nearby support group. If you have Internet access, alt.med.fibromyalgia, a Usenet newsgroup devoted to fibromyalgia, is a great place for information and support. This book also provides valuable information and pointers to useful resources.

DAVID A. NYE, M.D.
Midelfort Clinic
Eau Claire, Wisconsin

ACKNOWLEDGMENTS

My eternal gratitude belongs to my husband, Ed Hawes, for his unfailing love and support in sickness and in health—and in the writing of this book; the FMily, participants in FIBROM-L, the Internet fibromyalgia discussion group, who comforted me when I first joined the discussion, shared their lives with me, taught me what they knew, and cheered me on as I wrote; and Karen Boudreau, M.D., David Nye, M.D., and Elaine Turner, M.D., who generously critiqued the medical portions of the manuscript.

Thanks also to my agent, Nina Ryan, for helping me to find the right publisher and for her sound advice and encouragement; and to my editor, Jacqueline Johnson, without whose unfailingly gentle diligence a thousand things could have gone wrong that didn't.

Introduction

IN the autumn of 1993, I realized that I was barely functioning. My ability to absorb information was impaired. My work was taking me twice as long as it should. I could not remember a telephone number long enough to cross the room and dial the phone. I walked into furniture that had been in the same place for years, dropped things, and tripped over obstacles in my path despite having made a mental note to avoid them. I didn't dare drive a car; I was too accident prone. I had no choice but to see yet another doctor, although I had scant hope that the visit would result in relief for me.

But this physician was different. She nodded with recognition when I told her about my memory and comprehension problems. I mentioned the discomfort in my chest, a feeling of pressure around my heart and occasional shooting pains between my chest and upper arms. I told her I thought it didn't have to do with my heart because it was just as likely to occur when I was sitting quietly as when I was exercising. Standing behind me, she pressed places at the base of my skull, on my shoulders, back, and arms. I was surprised at how sore those spots were. Then she sat facing me and asked, "Are you sleeping?"

"I can hold still for eight hours, but my mind never shuts down," I replied.

"Do you dream?"

"No, at least not that I can remember."

"How many times do you get out of bed during the night?" the doctor asked.

"Five or six times," I replied.

"Do you wake rested?"

"Never."

"You're not really sleeping." Then she asked, "What's worrying you?" a question, I later realized, designed to assess whether I was suffering from depression.

"I'm worried that I won't be able to earn my living," I replied.

Then, for the first time in my life, I heard the word *fibromyalgia*. The doctor assured me that it is not life-threatening or uncommon. She told me the cause of fibromyalgia is not yet known and that it is therefore incurable, but its symptoms could be treated.

I was devastated. The notion that I had a chronic, incurable illness didn't fit my self-image of a strong, healthy, capable woman. The fact that fibromyalgia didn't threaten my life was not particularly reassuring. If this was what the rest of my life was going to be like, I'd just as soon be done with it.

I did what I always do when I'm confronted with new information that worries me: I headed for the library. There I found not a single book about fibromyalgia, so I drove to the nearest bookstore where I found nothing. I went home and turned on my computer, called up an information service I sometimes use, and searched available articles on any condition starting with *fibro*. I found an article on fibromyalgia and a couple of articles on fibrositis, which I learned was the old-fashioned term for fibromyalgia. What I read was a real eye-opener.

Fibromyalgia was the reason for my constant muscle aches and joint pains, and for the stabbing pains that from time to time made me catch my breath to keep from crying out. I found that the crampy diarrhea I had when I was younger was probably caused by fibromyalgia. I learned that fibromyalgia was the reason I could swell up like a balloon, gaining as much as five pounds of water weight overnight, usually losing it within a day or two. My poor coordination; the knee that sometimes forgot to catch my weight, landing me in a heap on the ground; the bursitis-like pain that a doctor once told me was all in my head; the sciatica that put me to bed for three months when walking became impossibly painful although my doctor at the time could see no reason for the pain—these things and many more were associated with fibromyalgia.

I concluded that I had had fibromyalgia since childhood. As a little girl, I was teased to the point of despair by schoolmates, teachers, and family for my clumsiness and poor coordination. When I told my mother about my aches she merely replied that pain was a normal part of living and that I should stop complaining. My adulthood was no better. After the birth of my first child I went to doctor after doctor, seeking relief for the pain in my hands that was so severe I had to use duct tape instead of pins to fasten my baby's diapers (this was long before the appearance of disposable diapers and Velcro fasteners). Doctors labeled me a hypochondriac and offered tranquilizers, sleeping pills, and psychiatric referrals.

After I finally received the correct diagnosis I learned that approximately 4 percent of the U.S. population—more than 10 million people, most of them women—have fibromyalgia. I found a fibromyalgia support group in a nearby city, then another, and another, until I discovered that five support groups meet within a twenty-five-mile radius of my home. I listened and learned, asked questions, got advice, and obtained references to medical papers, which I read with a medical dictionary by my side.

If I was so hungry for information on the state of my health, I reasoned, others must be, too. That is how this book came to be. I enlisted members of several support groups to become my interview subjects, to share with me their aches, pains, and ways of coping. I talked, by computer, with more than 700 people who subscribe to the fibromyalgia discussion group on the Internet, a worldwide computer network that schools, businesses, organizations, and individuals can join. (See Appendix A for more information on this and other resources.)

Throughout my research, I drew strength and sustenance from the people I interviewed. Two dominant themes emerged: People with fibromyalgia feel better, mentally and physically, when they can share information and support; and most people with fibromyalgia know more about how to cope with it than most health care professionals do.

Gaining support from others is more than a matter of listing your complaints and getting sympathy for your pain. Hearing from others with similar experiences validates you as a human being and improves your self-esteem. I had worked out several strategies to help myself deal with fibromyalgia, but I've learned many more ways since I've been talking with others who have fibromyalgia. This book will help you to do the same, whether you already know you have fibromyalgia or just know you suffer from chronic, undiagnosed pain.

I firmly believe in the adage that knowledge is power, and it is my intention that the knowledge you will gain by reading this book will give you the power to control, perhaps to overcome, the problems that fibromyalgia presents in daily life. You will read about the role of nutrition, exercise, and medications in making you feel better than you do now. You will read about nontraditional techniques such as meditation and visualization, about herbal remedies and nutritional supplements. You will find sources of further information, and of adaptive objects to make your daily chores and work easier. You will also learn a technique for troubleshooting your own case of fibromyalgia so that you can figure out what works best for you.

Between chapters you will find a series of interviews with fibromyalgia patients concerning their experiences in being diagnosed and treated, as well as the tricks and techniques they have developed to work around the symptoms that make ordinary work and home activities difficult. Names and other identifying information have been changed to ensure confidentiality.

By the time you finish reading this book, you will have a deeper understanding of the collection of symptoms called fibromyalgia. You will have a set of attitudes and techniques for making your life better at home and at work. You will have an arsenal of weapons to combat pain. You will know how to help your health care practitioner to help you—and have the courage and resources to find a new one if your present professional relationship is not working well for you. Most important, you will know that you are not alone, and that the discomfort you experience is *not* "all in your head."

A Cautionary Note

There is no one exactly like you anywhere in the world. Your body chemistry, your personality, and the experiences you have had in life are absolutely unique. People with fibromyalgia sometimes react strangely to common substances, particularly prescribed medications, but also drugs, herbs, minerals, and even vitamins. This makes finding what helps you quite difficult. You need to be careful, to try things cautiously, and to try one thing at a time.

I will not recommend anything that I know to be harmful or ineffective. Wherever I've heard that even one person has had an unpleasant experience trying something, I will say so, and describe what the unpleasant effect was. But you must use your own good judgment in deciding whether a technique or substance is right for you. (See the medical disclaimer on the copyright page.)

In chapter 10 I describe a set of techniques and procedures designed to help you experiment and find out what works best for you. Please, don't start experimenting until you have read that section. You'll find your results are far better if you approach the task of troubleshooting your fibromyalgia problems in a careful, methodical manner.

CHAPTER ONE

Fibromyalgia Basics

I F you're like most people with fibromyalgia, you ache all over and wish you could go to bed. When you finally get there, once your legs have finished twitching, you settle into a hazy half-sleep in which your eyes stay closed but you can't stop thinking. You wake up in the morning looking for the eighteen-wheeler that mistook your bed for the interstate.

Your energy level varies unpredictably from zero to two on a scale of ten. You lose your train of thought halfway through a sentence or—worse—throw in a completely inappropriate word that leaves you flustered and your listener baffled. Stupid things make you cry: a sentimental television commercial, a song you haven't heard since your freshman year.

You look healthy, in an overweight kind of way. You pass medical lab tests with flying colors. There's nothing wrong with you, doctors say. Knowing that you want a solution, they scribble something on a pad of paper and send you off to the pharmacy to buy drugs that give minimal relief, if any. Or they send you off to a psychiatrist. Or they tell you it's all in your head, and send you off in tears.

Fibromyalgia is most accurately classified as a *syndrome,* rather than a disease. A disease is a condition that has a known cause and can be identified by one or another set of laboratory tests. So far, we do not know of a single cause of fibromyalgia, and there are no tests that can make the diagnosis. There are, however, certain signs and symptoms that are characteristic of the disorder. (Signs are findings in an examination; they provide objective evidence of a problem. Symptoms are subjective and reported by the patient. They may not be sufficient to convince a doctor that anything is wrong.) A collection of signs and symptoms associated with a disorder is known as a syndrome. Fibromyalgia usually comes with a baffling variety of symptoms, which is the main reason so many people who have it may go without a diagnosis for years. Thus, fibromyalgia is often called the fibromyalgia syndrome, usually abbreviated as FMS, or just FM.

Signs and Symptoms

Fibromyalgia is a form of muscular rheumatism characterized by tenderness, soreness, pain, and muscle spasms. *Fibro-* means fiber; *my-* means muscle; *algia* means pain. Put them all together and they mean pain in the nonskeletal part of the musculoskeletal system—the muscles, tendons, and ligaments. Doctors used to call it fibrositis, and some still do, but that means inflammation of the fibrous tissues, an inaccurate description of the situation.

Most people who have FM experience aches and pains in their muscles most of the time, but fibromyalgia is more than that. The important thing to remember as you read the discussion of signs and symptoms that follows is that no two people experience fibromyalgia in exactly the same way. This makes it very difficult to diagnose, but there is one physical finding that is definitive. People with fibromyalgia have a sore or painfully tender feeling in some or all of the eighteen places shown on the diagram in Figure 1–1. The American College of Rheumatology (ACR) says that if you hurt when at least eleven of these eighteen tender points are pressed, and you ache all over, then you have FM.

Unfortunately, few medical schools teach the tender point examination in physical diagnosis class, and none taught it before 1985, so only those doctors who were graduated since then, or are interested in improving their diagnostic skills and have kept up with the medical literature, know how to perform this exam.

Table 1–1 describes these fibromyalgia tender points in plain English and in medical terms. Most are near the place where a muscle attaches to a bone. So far, nobody knows why this is so. You may not have all of these tender points at the same time, but if you have fibromyalgia you probably have some of them now, and have had others in the past. You may not even know they are tender until someone presses on them. The pressure need not be very hard at all to make them hurt. If your doctor says you don't have fibromyalgia without doing a tender point examination, ask for one. If the doctor flat-out refuses or says that it isn't necessary, find another doctor—one that will at least give you the courtesy of checking to see if fibromyalgia may indeed be your problem.

On the other hand, suppose your doctor does a tender point exam and finds fewer than eleven tender points. Someone who does not meet the syndrome criteria but has a typical history can be diagnosed as "possible FM" and a trial of treatment can be undertaken. Some who don't meet the criteria for FM probably have the as-yet undefined disease that causes it, but they also have a much greater chance of having some other disorder with superficial similarities, such as hypothyroidism or polymyalgia rheumatica. For these people, a much more extensive workup is necessary.

Another diagnostic criterion is the presence of pain in all four quadrants of the body—left and right sides above the waist, left and right sides below the waist, for at least three months. Thus, a case of sciatica (inflammation and pain in the hip and leg) or a case of bursitis (inflammation and pain in the shoulder), while terribly painful, does not in itself give evidence of fibromyalgia, even if you have both at the same time. But many people with fibromyalgia have had the pain associated with sciatica or bursitis, or both, without the inflammation.

Pain is not all there is to fibromyalgia. Disordered sleep afflicts about 75 percent (some researchers say up to 94 percent) of all people with fibromyalgia. People who have fibromyalgia

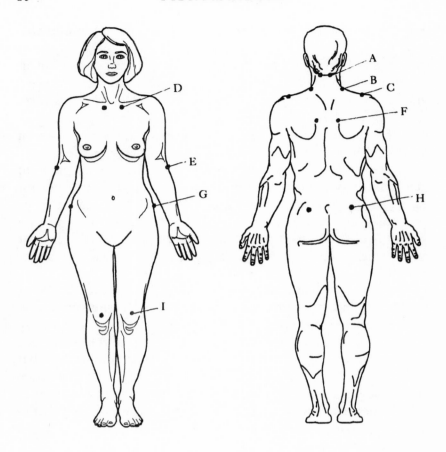

Figure 1–1, KEYED TO TABLE 1-1

usually report that they sleep lightly, are awakened by the slightest sound, and do not feel rested and refreshed in the morning. They can often fall asleep without difficulty, but as soon as they reach the deep level of sleep, they wake up again, usually remaining in a kind of twilight sleep all night. When they awaken in the morning, these people feel tired, achy, and stiff. Some people think this lack of restful sleep causes FM pain; others think that FM pain causes the lack of restful sleep.

Key to Figure 1–1	PLAIN ENGLISH	MEDICAL TERMINOLOGY
A	at the base of the skull beside the spinal column	suboccipital muscle insertions at occiput
B	at the base of the neck in the back	lower cervical paraspinals
C	on the top of the shoulder toward the back	trapezius at midpoint of the upper border
D	on the breast bone	2nd costochondral junction
E	on the outer edge of the forearm about an inch below the elbow	2 cm distal to lateral epicondyle in forearm
F	over the shoulder blade	supraspinatus at its origin above medial scapular spine
G	at the top of the hip	greater trochanter
H	on the outside of the hip	upper outer quadrant of buttock
I	on the fat pad over the knee	knee just proximal to the medial joint line

Table 1–1: DESCRIPTION OF THE FIBROMYALGIA TENDER POINTS

Whichever is correct, for most people with fibromyalgia, sleep plays a very important role in feeling better. I believe that sleep is so important in FM that I have devoted all of Chapter 2 to the subject.

Many of the symptoms that make up the fibromyalgia syndrome can also exist by themselves, without fibromyalgia. About half of fibromyalgia patients complain of either migraine or tension-type headaches, sometimes lasting for years and resisting relief from over-the-counter painkillers. About a quarter of fibromyalgia patients suffer from temporomandibular joint (TMJ) disorder, a painful condition thought to be related to the muscles and ligaments surrounding the hinges of the jaw, but not the joint itself. TMJ can cause terrible pain in the face and head. Some of the pain can be indistinguishable from that of a migraine or tension headache, but there is usually some pain where the upper and lower jawbones meet that betrays the fact that TMJ is involved. Closely associated with TMJ is the tendency often found in people with fibromyalgia to grind their teeth, especially during sleep, a condition known as bruxism.

More than half of the people with fibromyalgia suffer from irritable bowel syndrome (IBS). The most common symptom is crampy diarrhea that is often confused with colitis or Crohn's disease. But IBS can also make itself known by causing constipation, abdominal pain, abdominal gas, and nausea. Fibromyalgia can involve gastroesophageal reflux—a sour-tasting reverse flow of partially digested food to the back of the throat that people sometimes call acid stomach or heartburn.

Many people think the worst part of fibromyalgia are the memory and reasoning problems that often come with it. People afflicted with this cognitive dysfunction complain of being unable to remember things they have just been told, or to think a problem through to its conclusion. Others speak of "brain fog," a feeling that clouds inhabit the brain, that there is a fog surrounding them that keeps them from really being in the world.

Other symptoms sometimes present with fibromyalgia:

• Premenstrual syndrome (PMS) and painful menstruation

• Numbness and tingling sensations

• Muscle twitching

• Water retention and swelling, especially of the hands, feet, and face

• Dry eyes and mouth

• Dizziness

• Skin sensitivity, itching, and burning

• Impaired coordination

- Urinary urgency and/or burning

- Chest pain and pressure beneath the breast bone

- Intermittent hearing problems and low-frequency hearing loss

All of these symptoms can be triggered or made worse by weather changes, cold or drafty environments, hormonal changes before menstruation or during menopause, stress, depression, anxiety, and physical overexertion.

It is important to remember that having one or even a few of these symptoms does not necessarily mean that the diagnosis is fibromyalgia. But if you have low back pain and X-rays show no problem with your spine, and you have what appears to be a bladder infection and the tests come out negative, and you have aches and pains that come and go in various, unpredictable parts of your body—in fact, if you have any combination of symptoms described in this chapter, fibromyalgia may be the cause of your problem.

Possible Causes

Too little is known so far about fibromyalgia to allow researchers to identify a single cause. Without an identified cause (the medical term is *etiology*), no cure is possible. Chapter 6 discusses in detail what is currently known and thought about the possible causes and cures. This section provides a brief overview of the main theories. Any disease or disorder has at least one underlying cause. There is evidence that one or more of the following might cause FM:

• Metabolic dysfunction. Some researchers theorize that FM is caused by a problem in making use of or eliminating some substances within the body. Serotonin—specifically that too little is produced, or that it is reabsorbed before it gets time to do its work—is one suspect. There is also a suggestion that people with fibromyalgia do not excrete phosphates efficiently.

• Immune system disorder. Some evidence supports the notion that the immune systems of people with FM do not function correctly. There is suspicion that allergies, yeast infestation, and viral or bacterial infections may play a role in the onset of fibromyalgia.

• Heredity. There is strong evidence that fibromyalgia runs in families. Some relatives of people with FM have the clinical signs without the symptoms, and go through life without experiencing a fibromyalgia flare-up. Others have a full-blown case of it.

• Illness or injury. Many people can point to a specific incident that triggered their FM. Two common triggers are a case of flu and an automobile accident. Obviously, many people go through these experiences without developing fibromyalgia, so something else must be involved in those who do. Having inherited the predisposition may well be the differentiating factor.

• Prolonged stress. Whether it is physical—such as the need to wake up repeatedly during the night to tend a new baby—or emotional—for example, exposure to physical or psychological abuse—the bodily harm that results from unrelieved stress may be the underlying cause of many ailments, FM among them.

You can see that these possible causes are interrelated. For example, prolonged stress can compromise the immune system. It can also cause metabolic problems. Heredity may make some people more vulnerable to aftereffects of illness or injury. The possibilities for interaction are almost endless. Eventually, research will probably untangle this mystery. For now, it is up to us to figure things out as best we can.

It is sometimes useful to distinguish among three classes of fibromyalgia. *Primary* FM shows up early in life, with signs and symptoms emerging as early as four or five years of age. Children with primary fibromyalgia usually complain of random pains and aching legs. As you will see in Chapter 7, such complaints—often dismissed as "growing pains"—should not be ignored. There is growing reason to believe that FM in children can be reversed, if not completely cured.

Secondary fibromyalgia is associated with an underlying disorder such as hypothyroidism. Other sleep disturbances, such as apnea (a temporary cessation of breathing) and myoclonus (involuntary jerking of the limbs) are sometimes implicated as the triggering mechanism for FM. Sometimes middle-aged women develop FM during menopause, probably because insomnia is so often associated with this developmental stage.

Posttraumatic fibromyalgia has a clear precursor: an accident or illness. It can happen at any age, but its incidence increases with age. Most cases of posttraumatic fibromyalgia seem to be associated with a prolonged period of disturbed sleep, which may account for its appearance after a severe respiratory illness or accident involving severe pain.

We can eliminate the following as possible causes of fibromyalgia:

• Something toxic, such as exposure to a poisonous substance. There is no evidence that all fibromyalgia patients have been exposed to any such material.

• Vascular or circulatory problems. Many people with FM have poor circulation, but not all do, so this factor can safely be eliminated from consideration.

• A degenerative condition. There is no reason to believe that muscles, organs, or bones degenerate in fibromyalgia. Many people find that their muscles grow smaller and weaker from disuse, but that is true of people who do not have FM as well as those who do.

• Mental or psychological problems. Because people with fibromyalgia have so many different symptoms, doctors who don't know how to diagnose it often assume that the problem is purely psychological. These doctors are wrong, as clinical studies have shown. Fibromyalgia may cause one to become depressed, but depression does not cause FM, nor are its many symptoms imaginary.

• Tumors or growths. There is no evidence that tumors or growths have anything to do with FM. There is no relationship between FM and cancer.

A Brief History of Fibromyalgia

Fibromyalgia is not new; only the name is. Since the early 1800s, physicians have recognized and written about a condition involving disturbed sleep, fatigue, stiffness, aches, and pains for which there is little or no diagnostic explanation, calling it muscular rheumatism. In 1824, a doctor in Edinburgh described tender points. An American psychiatrist wrote in 1880 about a syndrome consisting of general fatigue, widespread pain, and psychological disturbance, and called it neurasthenia. He attributed it to the stress of modern life. In 1904, another doctor introduced the term *fibrositis* into the medical lexicon to indicate the sore spots found in patients with muscular rheumatism.

In a lecture published in 1913 in the *British Medical Journal,* A. J. Luff listed some factors causing fibrositis: He noted that symptoms in many people grow worse with the approach of rain and a lowering of barometric pressure, something with which fibromyalgics today are all too familiar. Extreme variations in temperature, local injuries such as those sustained in motor vehicle accidents, fevers, and infections of a flulike nature were also implicated. Dr. Luff drew a connection between fibrositis and the "growing pains" of which some children complain. He also blamed the absorption of irritating toxins from the gut as a cause of fibrositis.[1]

Perhaps because physicians would rather deal with an identifiable disease than an illness with many varied manifestations, fibrositis became a highly controversial diagnosis, and it has remained so in some quarters. More recently, doctors have realized that fibrositis is the wrong name. The suffix *-itis* means inflammation, and there is none of that in patients who complain of the symptoms of which we have been speaking.

Finally, in 1987, Don L. Goldenberg, M.D., published a paper in the *Journal of the American Medical Association (JAMA)*, reporting on the symptoms, laboratory findings and treatment results of 118 patients with fibromyalgia.[2] (He used the term interchangeably with fibrositis at the beginning of the paper, and stuck with *fibromyalgia* for the rest of it.) In an accompanying article Robert M. Bennett, M.D., wrote, "The term *fibromyalgia* has evolved from another with the same meaning, namely, fibrositis. Because fibrositis is a misnomer that carries a pejorative connotation, fibromyalgia, which sounds more scientific, has found favor with many physicians."[3] There was also an attempt in the early 1990s to rename the condition fibromalasia, meaning discomfort (malaise) in the soft tissues, but the medical community seems to be content with fibromyalgia.

Finding the Right Doctor

Despite Dr. Goldenberg's paper in *JAMA*, a highly respected medical journal, fibromyalgia still has a bad name in some quarters. Doctors don't like to give diagnoses that can't be proved by clinical evidence and, unfortunately research has not yet presented the medical community with a single diagnostic test that can prove the existence of FM beyond doubt. If you are confronted by a doctor who discounts fibromyalgia's existence because it can't be proved, you might want to remind the doctor that until the connection between the pancreas and sugar metabolism was discovered, doctors considered diabetes to be a psychological disorder.

If your doctor responds to your symptoms by acting as though you are an impossible complainer, or telling you that your problems are all in your mind, or saying that if you will only learn to control stress (or lose weight, or both) your pain will disappear, you may need a different doctor. If you had an automobile mechanic who told you the reason your car was stalling was that you worried about it too much, would you deal with that mechanic again? Surely not. You have a right to be treated with respect, and to have your problems approached with intelligence and concern.

But doctors do not always approach people with fibromyalgia, or with multiple seemingly unrelated symptoms, that way. They tend to dismiss your complaints and are less likely to see you as an intelligent, competent individual who would prefer to feel well.

A doctor's bias can have a profoundly negative impact on the quality of care you receive. People who have fibromyalgia tend to be overweight, possibly because their pain makes them less physically active than others, and also because of metabolic problems. Unfortunately, many doctors are prejudiced against overweight people, particularly women. This prejudice can obscure the doctor's ability to make an accurate diagnosis. Also, there are still too many doctors in this world who assume that most women's complaints are psychological in nature, and are apt to focus on depression as the cause of your problems, rather than as the result. I've talked with too many women who came to the doctor complaining of terrible pain and went home with a prescription for tranquilizers to recommend that depression be on your symptom list, unless the depression is threatening your life, in which case it constitutes an emergency that must be dealt with along with the physical pain.

One woman in a support group I attended told of seeing a rheumatologist at a prestigious medical center for two years without a diagnosis or relief from her pain and insomnia. She read about FM in a magazine article and recognized her symptoms. On her next visit to the doctor she told him she was sure her problem was fibromyalgia.

"I know that," the rheumatologist said.

"Why didn't you tell me?" the woman asked.

The doctor replied, "It's none of your business. And besides, there's nothing you can do about it."

In this woman's view, what was wrong with her body was certainly her business. And contrary to that doctor's opinion, there is a great deal you can do about fibromyalgia, even though there is no cure. Practically every person with FM has a bagful of doctor stories. Most of us have gone from doctor to doctor in hope of finding out what is wrong with us. Some of us have given up on the medical system entirely.

If you don't yet have a doctor who is familiar with fibromyalgia, there are several ways you might try to find one. You may know someone else who has FM, in which case you might ask about her doctor. Many communities have fibromyalgia support groups. There are more than 100 such groups in the United States. Often, a call to the local hospital will put you in touch with the leader of such a group, who may be able to give you the names of doctors about whom members have made good reports. Some support groups also maintain lists of doctors to watch out for, although this information may be harder to obtain. You may also want to call the Fibromyalgia Network (see Appendix A). This organization can give you a list of support groups in your state, and of doctors who have agreed to be listed as treating fibromyalgia. You should know, however, that the Fibromyalgia Network does not evaluate the doctors on its list and cannot promise a satisfying relationship with any doctor it names. When all is said and done, word-of-mouth referrals from satisfied patients are always best.

I found my doctor quite by accident. I had put off calling my HMO for an appointment until the situation reached emergency proportions, so I was given an appointment with the physician who happened to be on call that day. Lucky me. My regular provider had always been sympathetic when I came in with another symptom, but she obviously didn't have a clue that fibromyalgia was my problem and didn't offer much in the way of help. This new doctor recognized my symptoms immediately and I had my diagnosis within five minutes after we met. She gave me a prescription and told me to check in with her in two weeks. I thought I'd like her for my principal physician, but there were a few issues I wanted to discuss before I made the switch, so I set up another appointment.

At that appointment, I told her I was thinking of switching to her practice and asked her two questions. First, I wanted to know if she could tolerate being on a first-name basis with me. She said yes, certainly. Second, I asked if she could be my consultant while I made my own decisions. That was fine with her, she said. Her answers told me two important things: that she is not so impressed with her own authority that she can't tolerate a bit of informality, and that she recognizes that I know more about my own body than she does and respects my wish to be in control of its care. I was gratified when she told me that most of her FM patients knew more about the condition than she did, and she would be happy to learn from me as well.

The questions I asked my prospective new doctor may not be the ones you would ask, but I encourage you to think about what it will take to get you to trust the doctor, and make an appointment that allows sufficient time to conduct an interview.

You might find it helpful to have someone accompany you to the doctor's office. My husband went with me the time I was diagnosed with FM, partly because I was too accident prone to drive myself. Also, I was unsure of my ability to remember what I had to tell the doctor and I felt I needed an extra pair of ears to hear what she told me, and an extra brain to comprehend it. Any time you are feeling upset and shaky about your condition is a good time to take along a spouse, partner, relative, good friend—anyone you can count on to try to understand and be supportive.

If you cannot get anyone to go with you, it is especially important to list your symptoms and questions and take the list along into the examining room. Many people worry about being labeled as a hypochondriac if they come to the doctor with a list of complaints. This is not an unreasonable concern. Some doctors use the expression *"mal de petit papier"* (little piece of paper illness) in talking to their colleagues about people who come to see them with lists. One doctor told me, "Those of us who see a lot of FM accept this because there are a lot of symptoms to remember, one of which is poor memory, but this can cause instant prejudice in some physicians." Many good physicians have their patients complete a questionnaire before seeing them, in order to elicit symptoms that the patients may not connect with their main problem. If it does nothing else, bringing a list with you will help you to fill out the questionnaire.

If you suspect you have fibromyalgia, you might take the doctor an overview article (some are listed in the Appendix) and say something like, "I think I may have this." If you have underlined the symptoms mentioned in the article that apply to you, it also saves time and helps you list your symptoms without sounding like you are complaining.

Written information almost invariably helps. One person told me, "I have seen more than ten doctors and started a written summary after the third doctor. I found that this saves time and is easier for the doctor to digest when seeing a new patient. Here are the section titles that I use. I also update this every time I try a new drug or test."

> Symptoms
> Diagnoses
> Medications that don't work
> Medications that do work
> Therapy I have received
> Tests and a summary of results
> A list of physicians that I have seen

"Make each section brief and to the point," he suggested. "Keep all but the last item on one page. Make it easy to read—in outline form, for example. I always attach a copy of the results of any tests that have been done."

You may want to think twice about providing the names of doctors you have seen in the past, or at least omit those who you feel did not treat you with understanding and respect. Most of us have seen a great many doctors in the course of trying to find relief for our pain. Many doctors tend to be suspicious of new patients who seem to be doctor-hopping. They may think you are hard to get along with. Most doctors will listen to the opinions of other doctors in preference to those of the patient. If you give your new doctor the name of one who branded you as a hypochondriac, you may never get a fair hearing from the new doctor.

I would also hesitate to ask a new doctor for a painkiller that contains narcotics until the doctor knew me well enough to know that I don't take drugs of any kind unless there is no alternative. Some people go from doctor to doctor until they find one who will prescribe narcotics. Right or wrong, if your first request of a doctor who doesn't know you well is for narcotic pain relief, you risk being labeled as a drug seeker. A better approach is to list the pain-relieving medications you have tried, and the results of each. If the only thing that has helped is a narcotic drug, at least the doctor can see that you have tried other things. And there may be newer, nonnarcotic drugs available that your former doctors knew nothing about.

The point to remember, and to think of before your next visit to the doctor, is it is not your fault that you are ill. You have a condition that you didn't ask for and don't want. You are not to be blamed for not getting better. You have a right to expect that your doctor will not be patronizing or dismissive of you as a person, will not blame you for your troubles, and will listen with respect while you tell what you know about your own body.

If you have undiagnosed fibromyalgia, doctors can always tell you what isn't wrong with you, but many cannot tell you what is. And even among those who know something about fibromyalgia, many are not up-to-date on the best ways to treat it. That leads to one inescapable conclusion: You are going to have to help your doctor help you. You have an important role to play in making yourself feel better.

If this book does nothing else for you, I hope it will convince you not only that you must be in charge of your own treatment but also that you *can* be in charge of your own treatment. Taking charge does not mean that you make decisions on your own. But the doctor's role should be to help you understand what is going on and what your options are in dealing with it, and then, to help you implement whatever treatment changes make sense to you, including writing a prescription and monitoring your reaction to the new regimen. If you are going to succeed at this, your doctor must see you as a person to be reckoned with, a full partner in solving the problems that fibromyalgia causes.

Depression—Cause or Effect?

Many doctors tell their patients that their symptoms are related to stress or depression, but who wouldn't be stressed and depressed if they are in pain and deprived of restful sleep, as are many people whose fibromyalgia goes undiagnosed for months or even years? To be sure, fibromyalgia symptoms get worse under stress and depression, but making symptoms worse is not the same thing as causing them. Studies have shown that patients with fibromyalgia are no more depressed than those with other chronic, painful, and debilitating disorders, such as rheumatoid arthritis.

It is easy to see how a doctor could associate depression and fibromyalgia. Consider this very common situation: a patient, usually a woman, comes to the doctor's office complaining of insomnia and pain that seems to move from place to place, but is never completely gone. The doctor finds nothing in laboratory tests that can explain the pain and, knowing nothing about fibromyalgia, neglects to conduct the tender point test. Deciding that the pain is caused by tension, stress, or depression, the doctor prescribes an antidepressant. The patient's sleep improves (low doses of certain antidepressants are often an effective way to treat insomnia, a subject dealt with at length in chapter 2) and the pain goes away. The doctor feels completely justified in diagnosing the patient's problem as depression.

The fact that this doctor is wrong is not contradicted by the fact that nearly one-third of people with fibromyalgia have a history of depression prior to fibromyalgia's onset. For one thing, many people have fibromyalgia for years—in some cases nearly a whole lifetime—before they are properly diagnosed. Depression in the face of intractable pain is a logical response. Depression can cause insomnia, and a lack of restorative sleep can cause symptoms of fibromyalgia in almost anyone, and certainly in a person who inherited the predisposition to develop it. That is not the same as saying that depression and fibromyalgia are identical.

One fibromyalgia patient told me, "I think that we probably have a lot to be angry or depressed about—mistreatment by doctors, losing many of our enjoyable activities, having to deal with chronic pain and with people who don't understand it." One doctor told a patient, "With all the problems you're dealing with right now, you'd have to be crazy *not* to feel depressed."

CASE HISTORY: ROBERTA, 39, MUSIC TEACHER

On his fourth birthday, Roberta's son received a toy fishing rod and a cooking set. He decided to play camping, and invited his eight-year-old sister to play with him. Roberta overheard their conversation when her daughter offered to catch the fish for dinner.

"No," the little boy replied, "that's the daddy's job."

"Okay, I'll stay here and cook them," his sister said.

"No, that's the daddy's job, too."

"What can I do?"

The little boy answered, "You're the mom. You just sleep a lot."

Roberta recalls, "That was an entirely accurate portrait of the situation at that time. I was crushed, of course. I cried for a long time."

Gradually, Roberta did get better. Today, she is well enough to work as an elementary school music specialist. She sings in two choirs, has directed musical theater productions for both children and adults, and has recently completed an advanced recertification program to add regular classroom teaching to her music teaching license. But she still wonders what lasting impact her earlier dysfunction may have had on her children.

Roberta has had signs of fibromyalgia since childhood, although she has no clear recollection of pain as a child. However, she says, "I remember lying awake at night as a small child, feeling like I was going to explode or go crazy if I didn't wiggle. I get those same feelings now when I'm having a flare-up, if the weather is changing, for example, or if I stayed up too late. I must get up and walk around, stretch my arms. . . . Of course, now I know to go stand in a hot shower or sit in the tub to relieve some of those symptoms."

Now thirty-nine, Roberta was diagnosed with fibromyalgia about seven years ago. "I had become increasingly ill, new symptoms piling on top of old ones. Many were related to my menstrual cycle. I had multiple allergies, increasingly severe asthma, and premenstrual migraines that increased from one to eight days before my period. My PMS became severe, with anxiety attacks, fits of rage, and incredible mood swings. I had strep throat, bronchitis, and ear infections almost constantly. Finally, I started having chest pains," she says.

She found her way to a rheumatologist, who located her tender points and diagnosed FM. He told her, mistakenly, that fibromyalgia was a self-limiting condition that, in most people, ran its course and disappeared in one to ten years.

"By then I couldn't sit still, often having to leap out of my seat to pace back and forth. I felt as if my muscles were going to jump out of my skin. In addition, I had pains shooting up and down my arms, neck, shoulders, and back. I suffered great weakness, especially in my arms." For a week after each menstrual period, the muscles in her fingers would contract, turning her hands into claws and making it nearly impossible for her to hold anything.

During that phase of her illness Roberta put foam rubber handles on her hairbrush, toothbrush, spoon, and pencils. She bought a special pair of scissors, and gave up playing guitar and piano in her music classes, using instead an electronic instrument that played musical chords at the touch of a button. She took painkillers and antinausea medications for her migraines, antianxiety pills for panic attacks, nonsteroidal anti-inflammatory drugs (NSAIDs), and antidepressants for fibromyalgia; asthma medications; antibiotics; ulcer medicine for stomach pain caused by some of the pills; and something to relieve her heavy menstrual flow. "Basically, I was a zombie," she says.

Desperate for relief, Roberta took the advice of a gynecologist who said all of the symptoms were related to her menstrual cycle. She had a total hysterectomy. For the next four years, Roberta went into fibromyalgia remission. She had only a few migraines. Her hands were no longer contracted periodically, and her allergies and asthma improved. "Life got better," says Roberta.

Then her husband asked for a divorce. "He had had enough of taking care of me and everyone else. We went through intensive counseling alone and together for about two years before we both decided that we really did want to stay married," she says.

Despite the stress of a possible divorce, Roberta's FM was manageable during those two years. Since then, migraines have again become a problem, but she has stopped taking the NSAIDs. When her fibromyalgia flares up, Roberta's muscles seem to go into spasms when she stays in one position too long ("sometimes a half hour, sometimes two minutes," she says), and she must use her hands to move the affected part into another position.

Roberta has developed a strategy for sleeping: She makes sure she is asleep before her husband so that she doesn't have to hear him snoring. If that doesn't work, she goes to sleep on the couch. Roberta also has a tender point on her hip that sometimes acts up when she tries to sleep on her side. When her hip is bothering her she chooses the couch because it's softer than the bed.

Roberta's fibromyalgia has had a profound effect on her family life. Although her husband is still with her, there was a period during which he would become infuriated if Roberta had so much as a sniffle. "Over the past couple of years he has mellowed out somewhat," she says, "but I don't think he will accept and sympathize about any illness of mine, ever again."

It isn't any help that her interest in intimate relations has diminished greatly. "I don't know if it is caused by one of the medications I take, or by my lack of body esteem, but I have very little sex drive. For some time sex was the most repugnant thing I could think of. It's still not number one on my wish list, but I enjoy it more," says Roberta.

She grieves over the things she can no longer do with her children: roller skating and walking on the beach, especially when the weather is chilly. "Many times I have to say I can't do something they want me to do. I hate it," Roberta says. She worries about the model of adulthood she presents to her children, but has yet to explain her condition to them.

Most of Roberta's fellow faculty members know about her condition, although her principal does not. This is not Roberta's choice; the principal does not believe in getting too close to his staff, she says. "After all, he may have to make cuts, and it would be too hard if he knew our problems. Many of the faculty are friends who went through the ordeal with me. They watched me turn from a vivacious, hardworking person into a walking zombie who did minimal work. They also saw me climb back out of the pit." She believes in the wisdom of telling co-workers about her condition. "They need to know why I look like I have a hangover or am fuzzy around the edges if I have a sleepless night, that it has a much greater effect on me than it would on them. They may be tired, but they don't ache in every fiber of their bodies," she adds.

She usually has two major flare-ups each year, in the spring and fall when the weather is undergoing major change. Occasionally, she has other bad spells, usually as a result of overextending herself in some way. "I have experienced this many times over the past seven years: I 'forget' that I have FM, go back to being a night owl, work too long in the garden, and then I wake up depressed and in pain, completely surprised," she says. "I now just take this in stride. I know that I have good periods and bad periods. To me, the strangest thing is the 'amnesia' I have developed concerning my illness. I am always surprised by its recurrence."

Roberta's apparently indomitable spirit seems to work for her and against her. It is a gift to be able to forget the bad times—that's how Roberta gets as much enjoyment out of life as she does. But it is also highly desirable to remember the conditions required for those good times to exist. Roberta's spring and fall flare-ups are probably unavoidable as long as she continues to live where she does, but by modifying some of her activities, she might be able to avoid the lesser flare-ups entirely.

CHAPTER TWO

The Role That Sleep Plays

I F you are like most people, you spend about one-third of your life asleep. But if you have fibromyalgia, you most likely do not get enough sleep. How well you sleep is a major determinant of how well you live. Sleep affects how you feel both physically and mentally, how you behave, how well you can handle the ordinary stresses of life, how well you can get along with other people, and how happy and productive you are.

If you are not sleeping, you are apt to be cranky or depressed. You may be accident prone, a danger to yourself and others. You will find it difficult to think, to reason, and to remember. Sleep deprivation has been used as an effective way to torture and to brainwash prisoners of war and others.

Lack of sleep also compromises your immune system. When you are starved for sleep, you are vulnerable to the invasion of your body by illness. There is compelling evidence that sleep deprivation can also cause a significant amount of fibromyalgia pain.

If you have experienced insomnia or disturbed sleep for a long time, here are some clues to watch for in assessing your sleep problems. If your doctor dismisses your mention of insomnia or writes a prescription for a sleeping pill or tranquilizer without asking you questions about your wake/sleep pattern, you are not being treated properly. Be prepared to describe to your doctor exactly how insomnia affects you because this will make a difference in the diagnosis and treatment. Do you——

- have trouble falling asleep but once asleep, you remain so until the alarm goes off?

- fall asleep without undue difficulty, but wake up after two or three hours and don't get back to sleep until it's almost time to get up, if you get back to sleep at all?

- sleep but you dream almost unceasingly all night long and wake up feeling drained?

- believe you could fall asleep if your legs would stop jumping, or if you wouldn't twitch or startle just when you're almost asleep?

- believe you could sleep quite well if the person you sleep with didn't snore so much or so loudly or so irregularly; or if you didn't wake yourself with your own snoring, or because you're suddenly short of breath?

- remain dimly aware of your surroundings even while you're sleeping and can sit up and immediately take part in a coherent conversation if someone comes into the room?

- wake up more tired than you were when you went to bed, feeling as if you've been beaten or have the achy part of the flu?

You may find that more than one of these statements is true for you. Identifying the precise nature of your problem is an important first step toward solving it. Take time now to select those statements that apply to you so that you can help your doctor to help you, or perhaps help yourself without even needing to go to the doctor about your sleep problem. But most people with fibromyalgia need the aid of a health practitioner to deal with insomnia, because the most successful forms of treatment are available, unfortunately, only by prescription.

Individuals vary greatly in the amount of sleep they need. For adults, the average is between seven and eight hours, but that figure is nearly meaningless when you apply it to a single person. For some, five or six hours a night is enough; others need as much as nine or ten hours. But whereas there is great variation from person to person in the amount of sleep required, people's individual needs vary little from day to day once they reach adulthood. This is not to say that a person's sleep patterns don't change. In fact, as people grow older, they tend to sleep more lightly during the night and may nap during the day, which may make them even more wakeful at night.

The important thing to remember about the duration of sleep is this: If you wake feeling rested, if your alertness and energy during the day are satisfactory, then you are getting enough sleep. But if, as is more likely the case for anyone with fibromyalgia, you wake up feeling deprived of sleep and drag through the day in an irritable fog, then you have a sleep problem—regardless of the number of hours you spend in bed with your eyes closed.

Sleep's Healing Properties

Awake or asleep, your brain produces electrical currents that can be shown as waves on an electroencephalographic (EEG) machine. An EEG measures the average activity of the nerve cells in your brain. Your doctor may suggest that you have an EEG sleep study done to determine what kind and how much of a sleep problem you have. Most often, a sleep study is done overnight in a sleep laboratory, where you will probably bring your own pillow and be hooked up to an EEG machine. Sometimes a sleep study is done in the person's own home, in order to provide the most natural environment and study a normal night's sleep. Other times, the person is asked to sleep at the lab on two or more consecutive nights, in order to overcome the very common problem of trying to get to sleep in a strange place.

An EEG is completely painless. A technician dabs a bit of conducting ointment on some rubber discs that are attached to wires coming from the EEG machine, and places the discs at specific locations on your head. You will probably have been told to wash your hair before coming to the sleep lab, and not to use any conditioner or hair spray, which can interfere with the electrical connection necessary to measure your brain waves. (When you go home, you may want to wash your hair again to get rid of the residue of the ointment.) You will be asked to go to sleep as naturally as you can. During the night, the EEG machine will measure your brain waves. When your doctor gets the report, it will show how many times you woke up during the night, and how much restful sleep, if any, you had.

Sleep specialists speak of two kinds of sleep: REM (rapid eye movement) sleep and non-REM (NREM) sleep. Dream sleep is REM sleep; everything else is NREM sleep. If you watch a person who is sleeping, you can actually tell whether he or she is dreaming. Our eyes move when we dream, as though we were looking around. Our muscles would move, too, to mimic the motions in our dreams, if not for the fact that some nerve cells deep in the brain stem, the most primitive part of the brain, inactivate our muscles during REM sleep, making us almost paralyzed. If we move at all, our motions look more like twitches than actual motions. Most of us have observed this behavior in our pets, whose dream states are much like our own.

Some people have learned to put themselves to sleep by imagining that they are descending a stairway, going deeper and deeper into sleep. In fact, that is pretty close to what is happening. When you are awake, your brain cells fire independently, which is what makes the measured brain waves so short and choppy. The more you relax and the deeper you get into sleep, the more your brain cells fire in unison so that the recorded waves become slower, with longer intervals between their highs and lows. You go from a waking state through a phase marked by alpha waves, then into stage one sleep with slower theta waves. Next you reach the more rapid waves of stage two sleep; then, if you're lucky, you arrive at the blessed delta slow wave sleep, which lasts for about forty minutes in the first sleep cycle, and shorter periods later in the night (REM sleep occurs about every ninety minutes when we sleep). Dream cycles are shorter during the night and longer toward dawn. You probably dream every night, but you won't remember a dream unless you wake up from it. If you go right on sleeping, your dreams are forgotten.

Sleep researchers don't yet agree on the significance of the various stages of sleep. It is generally thought that psychological problems can result from the lack of REM sleep. Some doctors will tell you that it doesn't matter how much time you spend in any stage, or even whether you get to delta level sleep at all.

There is reason to believe that lack of delta sleep, leading to growth hormone deficiency, is at the heart of many of our problems as fibromyalgics. While the pituitary gland secrets growth hormone (somatotropin) around the clock, the largest spurt of growth hormone secretion—as much as 80 percent of it—occurs during delta sleep.

Most people with fibromyalgia get little, if any, delta sleep. Sleep studies done on people with FM have shown that in 90 percent of cases, alpha waves intrude as soon as delta sleep is reached. This is known as the alpha-delta sleep anomaly. This explains why fibromyalgics are such light sleepers, and why we can come fully alert if anyone comes into the room or speaks to us while we are sleeping. If we can't attain delta sleep, we cannot secrete enough growth hormone to meet our needs.

Researchers can get a good idea of how much growth hormone you have by measuring somatomedin-C, one of the substances left in your blood after the somatotropin breaks down. People with fibromyalgia have been shown to have less than the normal amount of somatomedin-C. It follows from this that we have insufficient growth hormone.

Growth hormone stimulates growth in children and adolescents, but it is important in adults as well. It is necessary for muscle health. As you move about during your waking hours, microscopic tears occur in your muscles. Growth hormone has a role in repairing your muscles. People with fibromyalgia tend to have muscles that are tighter and less flexible than those of most people, so we can infer that our muscles would be more subject to microtrauma. If we get more than our share of tiny muscle tears and less than our share of somatotropin, the result is the constant muscle ache and pain that is characteristic of fibromyalgia. Also, lactic acid and other substances build up in the muscles during exertion. Growth hormone helps in the process that carries these substances away from the muscles so that they can be excreted from the body.

A study has shown that many fibromyalgics can benefit from taking growth hormone, but so far the substance is prohibitively expensive. A warning here: This is not a place to treat yourself, even if you can obtain growth hormone outside the normal marketplace. An excess of growth hormone can cause acromegaly, a serious, disfiguring, and potentially fatal disease.

Anyone who is sleep deprived is subject to the muscle soreness associated with the lack of growth hormone. In 1975, Harvey Moldofsky, M.D., a researcher at the University of Toronto, Canada, induced the symptoms of fibromyalgia in healthy students by depriving them of deep sleep for three nights in a row. These students recovered promptly from their symptoms after a good night's sleep. (Fortunately, none of them was predisposed to developing fibromyalgia, it seems.)

Significantly, some students, all of them athletes, were able to avoid the FM symptoms. This is one reason why medical professionals who know about fibromyalgia urge their patients to engage in physical exercise as part of their treatment regimen.

Sleep deprivation has implications beyond the connection with growth hormone. There is some evidence that lack of sleep has a damaging effect on the immune system. Deep level sleep is vital for the production of antibodies, the chemical substances that neutralize or destroy the causes of most common infections.

Some people hear that the immune system may be involved and immediately wonder whether there is any relation to acquired immunodeficiency syndrome (AIDS). There is absolutely no connection between FM and AIDS. None. Fibromyalgia does not involve a weakened immune system and it does not make you susceptible to AIDS. Fibromyalgia can make you miserable, but it is not fatal and it is not communicable.

Fibromyalgics likely have hyperactive rather than immune-deficient systems. This would explain why many have chronic stuffy noses, multiple allergies, unpredictable reactions to prescription and over-the-counter drugs, and symptoms that change rapidly over time. Many fibromyalgics have red marks visible at the back of the throat that look like open and closed parentheses. These are known as crimson crescents, and are thought to be another sign of an overactive immune system.

One researcher found abnormal deposits of immune antibodies in the skin of a significant number of FM patients, suggesting that our cells allow substances to leak through the blood vessel walls and accumulate in tissues where they are not supposed to be. This could explain otherwise unexplained weight gain and swelling that so many people with fibromyalgia experience.

In strict scientific terms, the relationship between FM and immune system problems remains to be confirmed by more research studies. The scientific community does not usually accept something as fact until it has been demonstrated in more than one experiment. But there is little doubt that sleep deprivation does affect the immune system, and no doubt at all that people with fibromyalgia do not sleep well.

How to Get the Sleep You Need

Sleep disturbance associated with alpha-wave intrusion into delta-level sleep and insufficient serotonin are not the only causes of troubled sleep that may affect fibromyalgics. Most common among sleep-disturbing problems is a condition known as obstructive sleep apnea (OSA). If you sleep alone or with someone who sleeps very soundly, you may not know that you have it, and it may take a session in the sleep lab to determine whether you have OSA. It is more common among men. In fact, one estimate says that half of all men with fibromyalgia have OSA.

Our muscles relax when we sleep, including those of the

throat. As the throat muscles relax, the air passages narrow. If they narrow enough so that the walls touch, air passing through causes the walls to vibrate. Snoring is the result. In some people this narrowing is so extensive that the airway walls collapse completely. No air can get through, so the sleeper returns to a higher level of sleep; muscle tone increases, the airway opens, and the sleeper draws a breath. A rare form, called central sleep apnea, is caused by the brain's failure to regulate the muscles that control breathing.

If you are in the room with someone who has OSA you will hear loud snoring followed by a pause and a gasp. One person who suffers from OSA describes it this way: "When I fall asleep, once in a while I think my breathing stops. I get a choking sensation, as though I am trying to inhale but my throat has closed up. It is very scary. The first time it happened it became part of the dream I was having and I had one heck of a time waking up before I suffocated."

People with obstructive sleep apnea breathe intermittently when they sleep and therefore sleep lightly. As a result, they are tired during the day, just as a person with alpha-delta sleep intrusion is tired. And, as is true with any victim of sleep deprivation, the person with OSA tends to be accident prone. Falling asleep while driving or operating machinery is a real danger. People with OSA also have an increased risk of headache, hypertension, heart disease, and stroke. If you think you have it, you should consult your doctor immediately. It is readily treatable.

The most effective treatment for OSA is a device called continuous positive airway pressure (CPAP). You get a CPAP machine after a night or two in a sleep lab. Typically, on the first night your OSA is confirmed by means of an EEG to record sleep stages, plus tests for breathing patterns, oxygen saturation in your blood, and muscle activity. On the second night you are fitted with a mask over your nose connected to a machine that provides a little air pressure to keep your airway from collapsing. Once the pressure is adjusted to suit your needs, you may use the unit at home. A newer machine, BiPAP (bilevel positive airway pressure) senses when you are breathing and reduces the pressure. Sometimes nose plugs are used in place of the mask. These techniques work well for most people.

Another common cause of sleep disturbance is a bedmate who snores. This is a frequent subject for stand-up comedians, but it's no joke for the person who is kept awake by someone else's snoring. There are things you can do, however. Most snoring takes place when the sleeper is on his or her back, so anything you can do to prevent the sleeper from rolling into that position is likely to minimize the snoring. Some people prop a pillow behind their backs so that they are constantly reminded to sleep on their sides. One woman put two tennis balls into a bra that her husband wore backward to bed. Naturally, he woke up every time he rolled onto his back. Devices are sold that administer a slight shock or start a perceptible vibration in response to snoring. This may help the person whose mate's snoring is disturbing his or her sleep, but it is not a good idea if the snorer is the person with fibromyalgia. Disturbing that person's sleep still more is the worst possible thing to do. If you are a snorer who has fibromyalgia, you may want to ask your doctor to refer you to a sleep clinic or a sleep specialist.

Some substances can cause snoring and OSA. Alcohol, for example, is a potent muscle relaxant. People with untreated OSA should not drink at all. Some people snore only when they have had a drink or two. Some medications, particularly antidepressants, muscle relaxants, and seizure medicines taken at night, can cause these problems. Taking them earlier in the day may be a good option, but you should consult your doctor before changing the timing of your medications.

People who are significantly overweight sometimes stop snoring if they lose weight. Nasal problems—chronic congestion, a deviated septum, polyps, or allergies—can cause snoring and OSA. An allergist or otolaryngologist (ear, nose, and throat specialist) may be able to help. Antisnore pillows tip the head back to help keep the airway open. If you are the snoree rather than the snorer, industrial-quality earplugs may be the solution. Two antisnoring devices have recently come to market. One is an adhesive-backed strip that holds the nostrils open; the other is a U-shaped plastic device that presses on the septum, the wall between the nostrils. Both work for some people and are available at many drugstores.

It is rare for surgery to be required to correct snoring problems, and surgery is not as effective with OSA. Some people are helped by a device made by a dentist that pulls the jaw forward, or that keeps the tongue from falling back to cover the airway. The important point is that there are solutions to problems of snoring and sleep apnea. You needn't simply put up with having your sleep disturbed by either.

Bruxism, the grinding of teeth while asleep, is another sleep disturber. It is very common among fibromyalgics and may be a cause of TMJ (temporomandibular joint) pain as well as fatigue. Bruxism can be caused by psychological stress or abnormalities in the way the upper and lower teeth meet. Reducing the likelihood that you will grind your teeth in sleep may be a matter of reordering some parts of your life, learning techniques to manage stress, or getting braces on your teeth. Dentists can also fit you with a mouth guard to reduce the strain on your jaws and reduce the likelihood that you will grind your teeth at all.

Restless leg syndrome (RLS) and nocturnal myoclonus are two related conditions that can interfere with sleep, the former when you are trying to get to sleep, the latter when you have succeeded. If you have RLS, at times you feel that you just can't keep your legs still. This happens most often late in the day. If it happens when you are just about to fall asleep, it keeps you awake. I have this problem at times, and I've found a simple way of solving it: give in to the urge to move your legs. I move my feet rapidly, as though I were swimming with a flutter kick, for half a minute or so, several times with intervals of rest between. It usually takes three or four kicking sessions to get my legs to relax, but the technique has never failed me.

Nocturnal myoclonus involves sudden, jerking motions, usually of your legs but sometimes of your arms. This jerking may be enough to bring you up a couple of levels in sleep. People who have sleep myoclonus show a distinctive brain wave pattern on an EEG. Some people report that taking a calcium/magnesium supplement makes the jerking stop. Vitamin E (400 to 800 IU) may also help. If neither of these helps, talk with your physician. There are conditions other than mineral and vitamin deficiencies that cause this problem. An anticonvulsive drug may be in order.

Some common pain-relieving drugs may interfere with your sleep. A recent study found that aspirin and ibuprofen (Motrin or Advil) disrupted sleep by increasing the number of awakenings and the percentage of time spent in alpha-level sleep. Ibuprofen also delayed the onset of the deeper stages of sleep. Acetaminophen (Tylenol) was also tried, and did not seem to have any effect on sleep. Aspirin and ibuprofen are both classed as nonsteroidal anti-inflammatory drugs (NSAIDs), drugs that reduce inflammation and are often prescribed for arthritis for this reason. NSAIDs have been found to be of little help with the pain of fibromyalgia, which is no surprise since there is no inflammatory component to FM, so taking them near bedtime is probably best avoided.

Two common substances—caffeine and sugar—can also make sleep elusive and unsatisfying. If you have any trouble sleeping, you should give up caffeine completely—coffee and cola drinks are the worst offenders. Caffeine is a potent stimulant and it increases the tendency of muscles to go into spasm, something people with fibromyalgia definitely don't need.

If you do remove caffeine from your diet, do it gradually. Decrease your coffee or cola intake by a cup at first, stay at that level for a couple of days, then decrease by another cup and so on until you're done. Don't worry about how you're going to get going in the morning. You'll do just fine without caffeine, if you get off of it slowly. If you can't get up in the morning, it isn't because you have a caffeine deficiency, anyway. You need to work on your sleep problems.

Sugar is another matter. I'll have more to say about it later. But for now, you should understand that sugar acts as a stimulant (if you've ever seen a group of children at a birthday party after the ice cream and cake are all gone, you know what I mean), and you don't need stimulants when you're trying to get restful sleep, so don't consume sugar in the hours after dinner.

Other elements that can disturb your sleep include too much light or noise in the room, poor ventilation, and the wrong kind of pillow or mattress. Eye shades such as those given airline passengers on overseas flights can help with the light problem. If noise cannot be eliminated, you may want to try earplugs, or a noise-canceling machine. An inexpensive way to block out noise is to place a radio near your head, tuned to a place between stations where all you can get is static. Experiment with the volume until it blocks out other sound but doesn't intrude upon your consciousness. (Be sure you've found a frequency where there is no station in your area; you don't want to be awakened at dawn by a station that is off the air overnight.) Some electronics stores sell white noise machines that emit a sort of whooshing sound that many people find restful. There are also sound machines that mimic rainfall, ocean waves, bird songs, and other nature sounds. Ambient music, the kind used for meditation and relaxation, may also help you.

Mattresses and pillows are about as personal as you can get when it comes to preferences. Some people like water beds. If you order one, make sure it has a built-in heater, regardless of what climate you live in. Unheated water beds can get awfully cold in the middle of the night, and nothing bothers most people with fibromyalgia more than cold. If possible, before you buy a water bed spend a night at a hotel that has one.

Most fibromyalgics do well with a mattress that has a soft couple of inches on top and a firm foundation below. One way to achieve this is to place a firm mattress on a platform bed (or on the floor) with a three- to five-inch foam pad on top of it. Egg crate pads, the kind used in hospitals to prevent bedsores, are favored by some; plain foam pads work best for others. Before you use either kind, air it out in a sheltered location for a few days to let the odor dissipate.

Pillows should be capable of being compressed. Some people

like down pillows, or a down and feather mixture, but others are allergic to them. Nonallergenic pillows stuffed with cotton or a material that simulates feathers may be a solution. Many find relief for sore necks by rolling part of the pillow up and placing it under the neck, with the head on the rest of the pillow. Some people like neck rolls; others find that a towel, rolled and placed in a pillowcase, does just as well.

Deep, restful sleep is your best ally in fighting the effects of fibromyalgia. Do everything you can to improve the quality of your sleep. Maintaining a regular schedule that allows for sufficient sleep at the same time each night is especially important. You should have a going-to-bed routine that is relaxing and pleasant. I like to read in bed, although some sleep experts say this is not a good idea. I read short stories, so that I don't get involved in a novel that keeps me turning pages all night to find out what happens next. I play meditation music on a player that shuts itself off silently. I go to bed at the same time every night, with very few exceptions, turn out the light at approximately the same time, and get up eight hours later, usually feeling well rested, although I remain stiff in the morning from holding relatively still for so long.

One of the most important components in my good-sleep regimen is aerobic exercise. I ride a stationary bicycle for half an hour a day, six days a week. I take Sundays off so it doesn't feel like drudgery. Aerobic exercise, the kind that gets you slightly out of breath and causes you to sweat, is an excellent way of increasing your supply of serotonin. Studies have shown that exercise promotes sleep most effectively if you do it four or five hours before bedtime. If that isn't possible for you, do it some other time during the day, but do it. Walking is excellent aerobic exercise. I chose an indoor bike because I have no excuse if it's raining or the ground is icy. Low-impact aerobic dance is another good choice. Just be sure it's low impact. There are a number of excellent videos to help you establish an exercise routine. And if you can't exercise for half an hour, try doing it for a few minutes. When I started biking, three minutes was major exertion for me. I worked up from there slowly, increasing the duration only when the current level was easy. Do whatever you can, but do something. You will be rewarded for it, I assure you.

Prescription and Over-the-Counter Sleep Aids

To improve the quality of sleep, doctors commonly prescribe a tricyclic agent, usually amitriptyline (Elavil). People often resist the notion of taking a drug classed as an antidepressant, believing that it would label them as having a psychiatric rather than a physical disorder. In fact, tricyclic agents serve an entirely different purpose in the treatment of fibromyalgia than they do in treating depression.

Tricyclic agents work by delaying the reabsorption of the neurotransmitter serotonin into the nerve terminals, which is one way a neurotransmitter's action is stopped. Serotonin promotes sleep and eases pain, among other functions. Its products can be found in human blood and spinal fluid. People with fibromyalgia have been found to have smaller quantities of used-up serotonin than other people. It is not yet clear whether this is because our bodies make less serotonin or because our tissues break it down more rapidly. However, the action of tricyclics keeps whatever serotonin is available circulating, thereby making more of it available to promote sleep.

Like every other drug mentioned in this book, amitriptyline doesn't work for everyone. People with fibromyalgia often have atypical reactions to drugs. In addition to blocking the absorption of serotonin, amitriptyline does the same with norepinephrine, a stimulating neurostransmitter, so that some people who have fibromyalgia find that the tricyclic keeps them up, rather than helping them sleep. However, it is the least expensive of all drugs useful for inducing sleep, and its side effects (reduced libido, constipation, and increased appetite are the most common) may be preferable to sleep deprivation. Most people find that it reaches full effectiveness in about two weeks. As the body adapts to it, you may need to increase the dose.

Until 1990, when the U.S. Food and Drug Administration (FDA) banned its use, L-tryptophan was taken by people with sleep disturbances. An amino acid and a natural building block of protein, L-tryptophan converts into serotonin in the brain and provides good, restful, drug-free sleep when administered properly. The FDA banned L-tryptophan because a contaminated batch imported from Japan killed several people and left others ill. Although the FDA has known the cause of these tragic outcomes for years, it continues to ban L-tryptophan from over-the-counter sales. The substance is used widely in countries such as Finland, where no ill-effects have been reported. The ban is particularly puzzling since L-tryptophan is legal for use in infant formulas and in formulas for adults who must be fed intravenously. The ban is unfortunate, and an effort is under way in the United States to convince the FDA to rescind it. Many of the fibromyalgics I queried in preparing this chapter said that they would gladly resume taking it if they could. Tryptophan is available by prescription in Canada, where it is known as Tryptan.

I have found a substitute for L-tryptophan that works well for me. It is called 5-hydroxytryptophan, or 5-htp. It is a breakdown product of L-tryptophan and is legally sold in the United States by prescription, although it is not easy to find (see the Appendix for sources). It comes in 100-mg capsules; 100 mg of 5-htp is roughly equal to 1,000 mg of L-tryptophan. I take 400 mg of 5-htp at bedtime, sleep well, and wake up rested and refreshed. But don't take it just because it works for me. Talk with your doctor; provide him or her with the reference to 5-htp included in the bibliography, and then decide. If you do try 5-htp (or L-tryptophan, if it is available) you should take it two or three hours after your evening meal, and avoid protein foods (meats, dairy products, nuts) between dinner and bedtime. Washing it down with a glass of fruit juice enhances 5-htp's effectiveness.

Here are some other prescription medications to help you

sleep that doctors may prescribe. All should be taken only under careful medical supervision.

• Clonazepam (Klonopin) is an antianxiety drug that also has an anticonvulsive and antispasmodic effect. This can help relieve muscle twitching and bruxism. However, it can make FM worse if you don't have these problems, as it blocks deep sleep.

• Doxepin (Sinequan), like amitriptyline, is a tricyclic agent and an antihistamine with a strong sedative effect. It is often prescribed in conjunction with Clonazepam.

• Nortriptyline (Pamelor) is another sedating tricyclic, similar to amitriptyline.

• Tagamet (cimetidine) and Zantac (ranitidine) are normally thought of as antiulcer medications. However, they block the absorption of the stimulating neurotransmitter histamine, and appear to improve level-four sleep. They also increase the effectiveness of amitriptyline, and may be useful in reducing the amount of amitriptyline required, thereby decreasing that drug's side effects. A lower dose form of Tagamet has recently been released on the over-the-counter market.

• Paxil (paroxetine) is a specific serotonin reuptake inhibitor (SSRI). It seems also to produce its own pain-relieving effect. It should not be used with any other serotonin-enhancing drug. It is not a good idea to combine SSRIs with L-tryptophan or 5-htp.

• Alprazolam (Xanax) is an antianxiety drug that is known to increase slow-wave sleep. Its action is on neurotransmitter receptors, again making serotonin and other neurotransmitters more available.

• Carisoprodol (Soma) quiets the central nervous system. It should be tried in the smallest possible dose, probably half of a pill, at the outset and may be used along with a low dose of amitriptyline. It puts patients into a meditative-like state.

Some people have success with Benadryl (diphenhydramine), available over the counter in any drugstore. Benadryl is an antihistamine, an allergy remedy, but it also makes many people drowsy. If you try this, start with one 25-mg capsule and increase to 50 mg if necessary.

For people who cannot or will not take drugs, there are some nutritional alternatives. None of these has been subjected to clinical trials to prove their effectiveness, but not all of the drugs listed above have been scientifically proved to work with FM, either. These nonmedical alternatives are listed here because some people with FM are finding them helpful.

A good, yeast-free B-complex tablet in a high-dose—B-50 or B-100—has a calming effect on the nervous system. Be warned, however, that vitamin B_6, a part of the B complex, has a strong diuretic effect on many people and may cause you to get up to urinate during the night if you take it at bedtime. In general, vitamins are best taken with meals, preferably at breakfast or lunch. Herbal teas containing hops, chamomile, or valerian are sedative in nature.

Melatonin is a hormone secreted by the pineal gland primarily at nightfall. It is responsible for making us feel sleepy. Many international travelers and shift workers who need to sleep at unaccustomed times use melatonin. Doses for sleep range from 1.5 to 3 mg (a few people need 6 mg). Some find melatonin to cause depression; ask someone close to you to monitor you for signs of depression if you try melatonin. It is often difficult to detect depression in yourself until you are well into it and feeling so miserable that you can't think of anything that might help you. Melatonin is sold in some health food stores. It can also be purchased from a number of companies that sell vitamins by mail-order (see Appendix A). Large doses of melatonin (more than 50 mg) are being used experimentally for birth control. Women who wish to become pregnant should discuss its use with their doctors.

Some people get good results with a homeopathic formula called Calms Forte. Like the alternative methods just described, it is available at many health food stores.

CASE HISTORY: NAOMI, 45, SELF-EMPLOYED WRITER/EDITOR

Looking back, Naomi thinks she has always had fibromyalgia, but her symptoms became severe in 1986, while she was living in Hong Kong. When she moved back to the United States two years later, Naomi selected a new internist, the chief of staff at her health maintenance organization. She told him about her fatigue, chest pains, aches, irritable bowel, joint pain, and the shooting pains and terrible circulation in her hands. The internist referred her for consultation to a rheumatologist who "brushed aside my clipping of a *New York Times* article on FM and diagnosed me as an anxious hypochondriac," without so much as a tender point examination, she says.

When Naomi obtained her medical records to send to another doctor, she found the following in the rheumatologist's report: "No definitive objective findings to substantiate a diagnosis of connective tissue disease. It is likely that the patient's symptoms are in part related to her occupation as a medical writer and her general sophistication regarding medical matters, which has perhaps heightened her awareness of certain physical problems. . . ."

When her internist left the HMO, Naomi did, too. She visited the fourth doctor in two years, a rheumatologist who diagnosed her correctly, but prescribed anti-inflammatory drugs, an ineffective treatment for a condition that does not involve inflammation. She describes her reaction to being told there really was something wrong with her as, "relief and a sense of validation." Naomi says the diagnosis reassured her that she was not crazy, and made her furious at all the doctors who had dismissed her symptoms as imaginary.

Simultaneously, she sought help for seasonal affective disorder (SAD), a form of depression associated with lack of sunlight. The doctor prescribed light therapy and an antidepressant, both of which "helped a bit," Naomi says.

Aphasia, a deficiency in the ability to communicate through speech or writing, began abruptly in 1992. After several tests, a neurologist confirmed deficits but said they were due to "anxiety and my formerly high-pitched skills as a writer," Naomi says. Shortly after that, a psychiatrist told Naomi the aphasia was probably due to the antidepressant, and to unresolved issues concerning her failure as a fiction writer.

Naomi is sure the psychiatric labels in her medical record predispose physicians to dismiss her many symptoms and blame them on Naomi's emotional makeup. She has yet to find a doctor who will overlook the label of "hypochondriac" and take her condition seriously enough to treat her for it.

Naomi has most of the classic FM tender points. Some are exquisitely painful. She has remnants of bursitis in one shoulder and tendinitis in the elbow on the same side. Her peripheral circulation is so poor that she wears heavy kitchen gloves while scrubbing vegetables to protect her hands from cold water. Her arms go numb while she sleeps, or when she is sitting still. Naomi experiences irritable bowel syndrome. She is in the early stages of menopause, and is reluctant to blame fibromyalgia for menstrual irregularity. She has yet to find a prescription drug that will enable her to sleep soundly, or a doctor to prescribe it.

Naomi used to take great pride in being physically more adept and stronger than most women. "Now I can't do the fix-it chores and projects that I used to enjoy," she says. "I have to ask for help, which hurts me. I feel I'm not pulling my share of the load." Her husband is sympathetic to a point, and does not mind being asked for help. However, Naomi says he tends to accept the medical experts' judgment that she is a hypochondriac, abnormally obsessed with her own health and imagining her illness. "He openly resents the limits my fatigue and weakness place on our shared time, such as going out for the evening or spending the afternoon walking great distances. He also thinks I'm not trying hard enough to put this behind me. That hurts me deeply."

Fibromyalgia has heightened her insecurity over being several years older than her husband. "I have great fears that this aura of debility will affect his feelings toward me, make me defensive. . . ." She's aware of the danger that she might overdo it in an effort to keep up with him, "or risk his contempt if I admit to pain and limitations. This would surely undermine our marriage."

Some of the medications Naomi has taken have interfered with her sexual interest and ability to achieve orgasm. She has found others that do not have that effect, but pain is always a consequence of a sexual encounter. "I figure muscle pain afterward is the price I must pay, and I gladly pay it," she says. Her advice for people having trouble with their sex lives: "Adopt more passive postures, use pillows to support body parts as needed, and work a nap into the afterglow period."

Being self-employed has its good and bad aspects for Naomi. She can usually work at her own pace in her home office. "I'm not sure I could hold a nine-to-five job in someone else's office right now," she says. She has also equipped her office for her comfort, with an ergonomically designed desk and chair arrangement. She negotiates deadlines that leave time for unforeseen bad days. That means, of course, that she is earning less than she might without fibromyalgia, but she is more concerned with meeting deadlines than with earning every possible dollar.

Naomi has not told any of the editors for whom she works about her condition. She fears that they would see her as "a weakling complainer," which might cost her future assignments. Her difficulty in finding the right words when she is interviewing and writing is the worst part of fibromyalgia, as far as Naomi's work life is concerned.

Naomi is trying, so far with little success, to get help from a medical system that insists on seeing her problems as psychiatric in nature. The fact that much of her writing has been in the medical field may also be working against her. Medical terminology is a natural part of her vocabulary. Unfortunately, many doctors are still put off by patients who speak their language. It may be that Naomi's best chance at obtaining significant benefit from a doctor's visit will depend on her failure to make her medical records available, and "dumbing down" her language so that the physician can hear what she has to say.

CHAPTER THREE

Managing Pain

WE have all been taught that pain is a sign that something is wrong and that it must not be ignored. This is usually true but not necessarily when it comes to fibromyalgia. This raises two important questions: First, how do you know if the pain you are experiencing is FM pain or something else? Second, how can you deal with the constant, nagging pain of fibromyalgia?

The answer to the first question is not easy to find. Ask yourself this: Have I ever had this kind of pain before? When? Under what circumstances? Can I relate it to FM, or might it be something different? On one hand, if you can relate the pain to past episodes of fibromyalgia, then you probably need do only the things you do for fibromyalgia pain. You'll find some ideas for pain management later in this chapter. On the other hand, if you are not sure the pain is caused by FM, call your doctor's office, describe the pain, and let the doctor (or a nurse or physician's assistant) tell you whether it sounds like something you should make an appointment to discuss.

I have developed a rule that tells me when to call the doctor: If the symptom is new to me, and if I would call the doctor about it if I didn't have FM, then I will call the doctor even though I do have fibromyalgia. I'd rather live and be labeled a hypochondriac than die to avoid that designation.

Monitoring and Describing Pain

Many people find it difficult to describe pain to their doctors, perhaps in part because most of us have grown up in a society where bravery is highly valued, and to be called a crybaby is a great insult. If you are inhibited about describing your pain in detail, you must consciously change your beliefs about this. Only with a clear understanding of your pain can your doctor help relieve it, and you are the only person who can give an accurate description of what you are feeling.

One way to describe pain is by its intensity. Think of a scale of one to ten, where one signifies some discomfort and ten is reserved for the worst pain you ever felt. Beyond that, your doctor will want to know several other things.

• Frequency: Is the pain constant or intermittent? Do you feel it every day, several times during the past week, a few times during the past month, for example?

• Timing: When does the pain occur? Day? Night? Both? If it is recurring pain, does it begin at about the same time each day? If so, at what time, or during what activity?

• Duration: How long has this been going on?

• Rhythm: Is the pain constant, unchanging, steady? Does it vary or change in intensity? Does it just come and go? Is there any pattern that can help you to predict when it will occur?

• Accompanying symptoms: Do any other symptoms accompany the pain? Swelling? Nausea? Vomiting? Dizziness? Visual disturbance? Anything else?

• Description: Here are some words that describe pain. Use all the words that apply to your pain:
    aching
    blunt
    burning

cramping
dull
grinding
hot
inflamed
penetrating
prickling
pulsating
sharp
stabbing
stinging
throbbing

• Possible causes: Can you think of anything that might have caused the pain, such as overexertion, a fall, tension or stress, menstrual difficulties, or an injury related to sports or work?

• What you've done about it: What have you tried? What makes it feel better? What makes it feel worse?

• History: Has this ever happened before? What did you do then? What was the result? What seems to have caused it then? What is different this time?

The Many Sites of Fibromyalgia Pain

Fibromyalgia pain may take the form of deep muscle aches, burning, throbbing, stabbing, or shooting pains. Some people describe an aching pain deep in the bones. The pain may be constant, or it may come and go. It can attack one part of the body today and another part tomorrow, or it may pick its favorite places and concentrate on making you miserable in those spots.

Researchers have found that one of the characteristics that distinguishes people with fibromyalgia from the rest of the population is the presence of elevated levels of substance P in the cerebral spinal fluid of fibromyalgics. This appropriately named material is a chemical messenger that notifies the brain when a pain-causing stimulus occurs. It is not clear whether people with fibromyalgia have more pain because they produce more substance P, or that they have more substance P because their nerves transmit more pain. Substance P may have other functions as well as transmitting pain messages, but its excessive presence may mean that people with fibromyalgia feel pain from conditions that others wouldn't notice. This could explain why so many of us report to our doctors with pain symptoms that sound exactly like a specific ailment, but the results of tests for that problem show we are perfectly well. The pain we feel is real enough—it just isn't coming from where the doctor thinks it should be coming from.

Incidentally, if you smoke tobacco, you should know that fibromyalgics who smoke are found to have even higher levels of substance P than those who do not, probably making their perception of pain even greater.

In my experience, I have had pain that mimicked a gallbladder attack, when my gallbladder had been removed many years before; a herniated disc in my lower back, when X-rays showed no misalignment of my lumbar vertebrae; sciatica, when X-rays showed no reason for the pain; and much more. Most people with FM have been diagnosed with another disorder, such as rheumatoid arthritis, bursitis, or temporomandibular joint disorder, before being diagnosed with fibromyalgia. Some of them actually have these conditions; others have pain that is equally severe but only mimics the ailment. In 1984, rheumatologist Frederick Wolfe, M.D., surveyed a group of eighty-one patients that came to his clinic. He found that 12 percent had undergone spinal surgery, 33 percent had been hospitalized for low back pain, and 12 percent had been hospitalized for neck pain. Dr. Wolfe blames the high rate of hospitalization on the failure of many doctors to recognize FM. Only 6 percent of the fibromyalgia patients seen in his clinic come in with the correct diagnosis.

This does not mean that people with FM never have any of the disorders that fibromyalgia pain can mimic. But it does mean that if testing shows you don't have the disorder the doctor suspected, the doctor should suspect fibromyalgia and do a tender point exam on the spot.

Muscle Pain

Muscle pain is common in fibromyalgia. Many of us hold our muscles so tightly that they are prone to go into spasms. Take me, for example: I am definitely not a tense person. With a good deal of time and perseverance, I have learned to take most things in stride. Sometimes pain may get to me and make me cranky, but I rarely get angry—it's hardly ever worth the energy cost. But I have noticed that when I lie down at night to go to sleep, if I don't concentrate on relaxing each muscle group individually, my muscles are as taut as guitar strings. Sometimes I wake in the middle of the night, my body so tense that I might as well be trying to levitate. Even my face muscles are tensed.

What about you? Right now, where are your shoulders in relation to your ears? How would you describe the position of your eyebrows? How tight is your jaw? How taut are the muscles of your legs and buttocks? As with most people with fibromyalgia, you may be in a serene state mentally, but your body just doesn't get the message.

Walking around all day with your muscles pulled up tight is an excellent way to cause pain. I've been working for months on becoming more aware of my muscle tension. Biofeedback may help you, but sometime you'll have to turn off the biofeedback machine, so here is a method you can use anywhere. Set a timer or wristwatch alarm to alert you every hour—or whatever is convenient for you—and when it goes off, run your checklist.

- Face
- Jaw
- Shoulders
- Arms
- Buttocks
- Legs

All parts of your body should be relaxed, though not limp, your head settled comfortably above your spinal column. Take a couple of slow, deep breaths and go back to what you were doing, being sure that your alarm will remind you to check for tenseness an hour later.

Cold temperatures are a major cause of muscle spasms. Keep yourself warm. If you live in a cold climate, dress in layers so that you can take a garment off or put one on as the temperature around you changes. Even in summer, I carry a sweater when I go out if there's any chance I may find myself in an air-conditioned place.

Abnormally tight muscles are at greater risk for the tiny tears in muscle fiber that occur during the course of a normal day's work. Normally, these microtears are repaired during sleep, but if you're not getting restorative sleep, repairs are not made and soreness results.

Two nutritional supplements may help with muscle pain and spasm. Many people report that magnesium supplementation helps. You can find magnesium tablets at a health food store and in many pharmacies. Magnesium tends to cause diarrhea in some people, so start with a small dose—say half a tablet—and work up to a full dose after you have had a few days to see how it affects you. Another idea is to take a calcium/magnesium supplement. Calcium is good for muscle tone, and has the opposite effect to magnesium on your digestive system. Vitamin E (400 to 800 IU) may also help with muscle cramps and spasms. Unlike water-soluble vitamins, whose excess is excreted in the urine, minerals and oil-based vitamins (A, D, and E) do build up in your system and can cause toxicity. Don't believe that if some is good, more is better. Finally, some people experience relief from muscle stiffness by taking 500 mg each of the amino acid supplements L-arginine and L-lysine. (Lysine is regularly added to cattle feeds to build strong muscles in animals raised for food.)

Back and Neck Pain

Probably nothing compares with back pain when you're trying to get anything done at work or around the house. Pain in the back and spine is one of the most common complaints of people with fibromyalgia. The pain may be caused by FM, or it may be the triggering cause of FM by interfering with sleep. Back pain is easier to prevent than to cure, so this discussion starts with some suggestions for avoiding it. Before you decide to do anything about your back, you should see your physician and rule out pinched nerves or a herniated disc, medical conditions that may require more than the measures discussed here. But even if you have a medical problem with your back, you should ask if these techniques are appropriate for you.

The way you sit, stand, and pick things up can determine whether you will suffer from pain in your back. If you sit at a desk all day, insist on a good chair, one that supports you, is the right height, and is comfortable. Get a chair with arm rests, if possible. Stand up as often as you can to find a file, get a drink, and so forth. If your hands are on a keyboard much of the time, sit so that your forearms are parallel with the floor. If you often feel pain across your shoulders, your seat is too low and you are reaching up to the keyboard or desktop. Get a wrist support or roll up a small towel to put under your wrists at the keyboard. Put a phone book, door mat(s), or footrest under your feet so that your thighs are parallel to the floor. If your chair does not have a built-in lumbar (lower back) support, make a lumbar roll to ease the pressure on nerves in the lower back and retain the curve in your lower back. An easy way to do this is to roll up a hand towel and place it behind the small of your back, then scrunch your buttocks as far back in the seat as you can. Whether or not you use a lumbar roll, cultivate the habit of sitting as far back in any chair as possible. An easy way to keep the roll with you at all times is to put it in a waist pack and wear it. I did this for two years until I got my lower back feeling fine. I still do it on long drives, especially when I'm the driver. If you prefer to buy a ready-made lumbar roll, you'll find a source in Appendix A.

Sciatica is a painful condition characterized by pain in the hip that radiates down the leg and into the foot. The farther toward your foot the pain travels, the worse the condition is and the longer it is likely to persist. One common cause of sciatica is a spasm of the piriformis muscle, which extends from the sacrum at the end of the spine to the hip joint. If you feel pain in your hip, please don't ignore it. I did for the better part of a year, and spent four months in bed as a result. (There is a school of thought that says a few days of bed rest can be beneficial, but people recover faster if they don't stay in bed. However, if the pain you experience when trying to walk is unbearable, bed is the only option.) Now that I know what to do when a muscle spasm begins, I have had no trouble with my back, or with sciatica, for six years.

Here's what I learned from a wise and patient physical therapist: If your back begins to hurt—or, better, if you've engaged in work or exercise that may have put a strain on your back muscles—lie face down on the floor immediately with your hands by your sides and your head turned to one side. (If your head won't turn that far, put a small rolled towel or pillow under your chin and rest your chin on it.) If the pain is more severe on one side than the other, shift your hips a few inches *away* from the pain. Concentrate on relaxing, particularly the muscles of your back and legs. If you don't make your muscles relax, this technique will not work. Stay this way for five minutes or more, then raise your upper body by placing your hands under your shoulders and leaning on your forearms. Stay this way for five minutes or more, always focusing on the relaxation of your back and leg muscles. Then, still keeping your back muscles relaxed, try to straighten your arms so that your back arches. Hold this position for a couple of seconds and get back down on your forearms. Repeat this motion several times, each time trying to get your arms a little bit straighter, while being sure that your back, hip, and leg muscles are relaxed and your pelvis is on the floor. If your pain is great, you should do this routine every couple of hours.

These exercises and more can be found in *Treat Your Own Back*, by Robin McKenzie (see Appendix A). Do the exercises anytime you feel pain starting in your back and as a preventive measure whenever you have been engaged in lifting or bending over.

Applying ice to your lower back is another way to get relief. I have iced both my knees and (with help) my low back/tailbone area with considerable success. The technique can work on almost any part of the body where musculoskeletal pain is involved. My physical therapist taught me to do it this way.

- Freeze water in individual paper cups, either bathroom size or one size larger. Tear off the first inch or two of the cup, leaving the bottom and lower sides on the ice to give you something to hold on to.

- Rub the ice lightly in a circle, the circumference of which is wider than the painful area, with the most painful part in the center. Keep the ice moving slowly in a circle, covering the entire area, for about ten minutes. Do not press on the area, just touch it with the ice.

- When the center of the circle begins to turn pale, it's time to stop. You can repeat this every three to four hours if it helps.

In addition to numbing the immediate area (cold nerves don't convey pain impulses efficiently), this technique releases pain-relieving endorphins in your brain.

I have also used a form of pelvic traction. It requires that you have enough strength in your arms to hold your weight for a few minutes, and shoulders that will allow you to get your arms and hands up over your head, so it is not for everyone. I use a chinning bar, firmly secured in a doorway. Exactly how high you place the bar depends on your height, and how far you can extend your arms. I grip the bar and bend my knees, raising my feet off the floor and allowing the weight of my lower body to pull on my spine. I do this as long as I can before the strain starts to hurt my shoulders, usually only a minute or two at a time. It's very important to be sure that the bar is firmly fixed, so it won't fall while you're hanging from it, or you could be seriously injured.

Neck pain is also common among people who have fibromyalgia. In some, tight neck muscles, usually a response to pain, cause the cervical (neck) vertebrae to lose their natural curve, sometimes causing nerves to be pinched. Much shoulder pain actually comes from a misalignment of the cervical vertebrae. *Treat Your Own Neck* by Robin McKenzie, a companion book to the one mentioned above, contains exercises and many ideas for relieving neck pain. One of its suggestions is that you place a pillow roll under your neck when you sleep. Cervical pillows are also available, and many people with neck problems find them a great relief. Devices for cervical traction to be used at home are also available. They are reasonably inexpensive and hang on a door. You should check with a physician or physical therapist before using cervical traction; necks are complex structures and a neck injury can be serious.

If your back is bothering you, here is a way to get out of bed that won't make things worse. Roll onto your side close to and facing the edge of the bed. Draw your knees up, then drop your feet over the side of the bed; use your arms to push yourself up, and roll into a sitting position. It won't be painless, but it's a lot better than using your abdominal and back muscles to help you to sit up.

Foot Pain

Sciatica also can cause pain in the foot, as well as in the hip and leg. The foot pain I experienced when I had sciatica felt as though I were standing barefoot on the rung of a ladder, with my weight on the arch of my foot. I also at times felt as though my two or three smallest toes were tied up by a piece of twine that was being drawn tighter and tighter. I had these feelings for quite a while after the sciatica was almost gone and I was working once again. It seemed to be worse when I had been sitting for a long while, and I learned that I could get some relief by standing up and arching my back.

Another kind of foot pain common in fibromyalgia is called plantar fasciitis—an inflammation of the connective tissue (fascia) that lines the sole of the foot. The main symptom is pain in the sole of the foot, especially at the front edge of the heel. The pain is usually the worst when you first get out of bed in the morning. Some people get relief from nonsteroidal anti-inflammatory drugs (NSAIDs) such as aspirin, ibuprofen, or naproxen. Doctors sometimes give local anesthetic or cortisone injections in the inflamed area. Applying ice packs three or more times a day may help. Some people tape the arch of the foot, using athletic type adhesive tape. Start at the top of the foot, run the tape around under the arch and back up to the top of the foot, stopping an inch or so from where the tape was first attached, applying mild tension. The purpose is to keep your arch from flattening completely when you step on that foot. Use three strips of tape, slightly overlapping. *Do not make a complete loop around the foot* because that could cut off blood circulation and cause worse problems.

The best help for plantar fasciitis is a pair of custom-made orthotics—inserts for your shoes that are made from plaster casts of your feet. They are often made of leather (for the part that touches your feet) and a fairly firm polyfoam. It takes time to get used to them, but the effort is worthwhile. Orthotics are not cheap, but if your doctor prescribes them, you may be able to get reimbursement from your health insurance. If orthotics are out of the question, go to the foot-care section of any large drugstore and look for arch supports.

If your pain is in the ball of your foot exclusively, you may have fallen metatarsal arches (the arch that runs the length of the ball of your foot from the base of your toes to the big transverse arch). You can buy metatarsal arch supports; they feel like marbles in your shoes for the first few days, but once you get used to them, they are a great relief.

Chest Pain

Chest pain caused by fibromyalgia is tricky. It can make you think you are having a heart attack, and if you have the least suspicion you are having cardiac distress, you should call your doctor or go to the nearest hospital emergency room immediately! Don't be embarrassed if you do this and find out there's nothing wrong with your heart. It's certainly better to be over-cautious than neglectful in this case. In time you will learn to recognize FM-related chest pains.

The most common cause of FM chest pain is a condition called costochondritis. There is a place in the chest where the ribs turn to cartilage and attach to the breastbone (sternum). These attachments, which are directly over the heart, can become sore and inflamed, mimicking angina pectoris, the chest pain that results from the muscle wall of the heart being temporarily deprived of oxygen. To complicate matters, if the pain of costochondritis frightens you, you may begin pumping adrenaline as you would with any other fright, making your heart race and adding to the impression that you are having a heart attack.

Sometimes chest pain is caused by tender points or trigger points (see Chapter 5) in the pectoral (chest) muscles. You may be able to feel around and find the spot that is causing the pain. If pressing on it makes the pain worse, you've found the right place. Gently but firmly rubbing or stretching those muscles may bring relief.

Some doctors treat FM-caused chest pain by injecting a local anesthetic such as lidocaine into the area. The pain should disappear within seconds if tender points, trigger points, or costochondritis is the culprit.

Sharp pains in the chest that move from place to place are probably caused by digestive gasses. But, again, if you are not sure, seek medical advice.

Hand Pain

Carpal tunnel syndrome (CTS) is the cause of much pain in people who have fibromyalgia. In fact, it is sometimes the trigger that causes a person to develop FM by interfering with restful sleep. The pain, which is caused by compression of a nerve in the wrist, is often felt in the fingers or lower arm as well. Sometimes the fingers turn numb. A doctor can diagnose CTS by means of a test called an electromyogram (EMG), in which needles are inserted to determine whether nerves are supplying messages to the muscles. True carpal tunnel syndrome is usually treated by wearing wrist splints to relieve pressure on the nerve and allow it to heal. Sometimes surgery is required to enlarge the space in the wrist bones through which the nerve passes.

Quite often, an EMG test done on a person with fibromyalgia who is suffering from severe wrist and hand pain shows no carpal tunnel involvement. If this happens to you, here is a suggestion that may help you to find relief. Take vitamin B_6. This has never been tested in a clinical setting, so there is no scientific evidence that it works, but many who have tried it say it works for them, and it certainly worked for me.

Deficiencies of B vitamins (specifically B_6) are suspected of causing swelling of the nerves, as well as other nervous and emotional symptoms. Some nutrition experts believe that the ability to absorb nutrients, including B vitamins, from food is compromised in people with fibromyalgia. Therefore, there is a possibility that what appears in fibromyalgics to be carpal tunnel syndrome is really a swelling of the nerve, resulting in pain and numbness of the hand, wrist, or forearm.

This was true in my case, and it was also true of much of the pain I had in my shoulders at the same time. I took a large dose of vitamin B_6 for three weeks—100 mg per day, half at breakfast and half at lunch. (B_6 can act like a diuretic in some people, so I don't advise taking it at bedtime.) The results in my case were startling; the release from pain was complete. This has not worked every time for me since then, but it has worked enough times that I recommend it for people who seem to have CTS but don't test out that way.

I stress the three-week part of the suggestion because if you take large doses of any one B vitamin for too long you may cause deficiencies in the other B vitamins. They don't call it B complex for nothing. If the B_6 works and you want to continue, then after three weeks you need to replace it with a B-100 tablet, which contains 100 mg of B_6 and proportional amounts of the other Bs. If it doesn't work after three weeks, it probably never will.

It is unlikely you can do any harm trying this method. B vitamins are water soluble; what you don't need you excrete in your urine. There was a widely publicized story a few years ago about a man who became toxic taking B vitamins; symptoms included stumbling, mumbling, and other indicators of neurological involvement. This was supposed to be a warning to people not to take more than the recommended daily allowance of B vitamins; 100 mg of B_6 is a great deal more than that. What the news stories didn't tell was that the man was taking six *grams* (the equivalent of sixty B-100s) a day, and that his symptoms disappeared within forty-eight hours after he stopped taking them.

Headaches and Migraine

Headaches are common in the general population; one source says that one out of ten people suffers at least one headache a week. But they are far more common among people who have fibromyalgia. A 1990 estimate said that nearly 53 percent of fibromyalgics list headaches as one of their major problems. Most headaches are associated with swelling or inflammation of blood vessels in the head. Causes may be tension, fatigue, tight neck muscles, or sinus or other infection, to name a few. You can usually identify a sinus headache: You probably have had a cold recently, or you have been exposed to something to which you are allergic. Sinus headache pain is usually worse around and behind the eyes. If you bend over or change altitude—in an airplane, for example—the pain gets worse. A headache that lasts for a long time can be a sign of something worse. If you have a headache that just won't quit, you should see a doctor to be sure it's nothing serious.

Migraine is a particularly severe type of headache. It usually causes intense, throbbing pain, usually on one side of the head, the forehead, or the temples. A migraine can last for several hours or several days. It is often accompanied by extreme sensitivity to light and sound, dizziness, nausea, and vomiting. Certain foods, including chocolate, bananas, nuts, and alcoholic drinks, can trigger migraine. Women with migraine outnumber men by about three to one; hormonal changes often cause migraine, particularly in association with menstrual periods. NSAIDs and over-the-counter drugs such as acetaminophen help some headaches. Migraine may require prescription drugs or, in extreme cases, injections, some of which you can administer yourself with a device much simpler to use than a hypodermic needle. If headaches are a major problem for you, you should probably see your health care provider for advice. If they are only a sometime nuisance, the following suggestions may help.

• Drink lots of fluids. Water is fine for the purpose; fruit juices may contain too much sugar, which only makes things worse in the long run.

• Especially if it's a sinus headache, try steam. Pour boiling water into a large bowl. A couple of drops of eucalyptus oil will help clear up congestion in your head and chest, if that's a problem. Bend your head over the bowl—be careful not to burn yourself with the steam—and use a towel to make a tent so that the steam stays inside. Breathe as deeply as you can, and try to relax.

• An ice pack, either on your forehead or the back of your neck, sometimes helps. Try alternating steam with ice packs.

• Put your thumb on the fleshy pad at the base of your thumb and your forefinger on the back of your hand opposite your thumb and press hard. If you do this when you have the first hint of a headache, it may go away entirely.

• Watch what you eat. If headaches are a continuing problem for you, keep a food diary for a week, noting what you eat, the time of day you ate it, and the time of day your headache started. You may see a pattern. Be especially suspicious of anything containing refined sugar. Chocolate and nuts are also often to blame.

Facial Pain

Temporomandibular joint disorder (TMJ, or TMD) is a common problem among people who have fibromyalgia. The temporal bone in your skull is the big bone behind your temple; the mandible is your lower jaw. Where these two come together is a kind of hinge called the temporomandibular joint. If this joint doesn't work smoothly, it can cause a lot of pain.

One possible cause of TMJ pain is the tendency of many fibromyalgics to grind their teeth during sleep, and even sometimes when they are awake. The tightness of our muscles often makes us clench our jaws, putting undue strain on the joint. Missing teeth, especially toward the back, and upper and lower teeth that don't meet properly (a condition known as malocclusion) can contribute to TMJ.

The pain can be truly terrible, but there are things that can be done. If you grind your teeth, your dentist can fit you with a mouth guard something like those that football players wear, to keep you from putting stress on your jaw when you sleep. A dentist also may be able to correct your bite to minimize or eliminate the malocclusion.

There are also things you can do to help yourself. Because I tend to clench my jaw, I have cultivated the habit of keeping my tongue forward in my mouth, touching the backs of my upper teeth. If you were to look at me, you wouldn't notice this, but when I start to clench my jaws, I get immediate feedback (I bite my tongue). I don't have much trouble remembering not to clamp down anymore.

Another technique is to pay attention to your posture, keeping your head on top of your spinal column. Don't look down when you're eating, talking, or singing. Looking down forces your lower jaw forward, and possibly out of place.

If your lower jaw feels like it is out of place, here's a little exercise that may help get it back where it belongs. Put your thumbs behind both upper canine or eye teeth (left thumb behind left eye tooth, right thumb behind right eye tooth), consciously make your jaw relax, and pull gently forward. Hold this position for one minute; do this frequently. The effect is to make the temporomandibular joint slip into its natural position. (If you work in an office where co-workers can see you, a little explanation may be in order.)

Medicines for Pain Relief

One of the trickiest problems facing people with chronic pain is knowing when to try to tough it out and when to take some form of medication for relief. What works for me also may help you.

For most of my life, I have had some level of pain every day. Gradually I managed to reduce my pain to the level of background noise—something like the street noise, or the sounds of the office where you work, that you grow accustomed to and filter out of your consciousness. Much of the time, this works.

Sometimes, however, the pain demands my attention. When that happens, I don't hesitate to seek relief. I've learned that certain kinds of pain simply won't go away until I throw some kind of pain medicine at them—muscle spasms, particularly in my back or hands (because I spend my days typing on a keyboard), and headaches are particularly hard for me to get rid of once they take hold.

For back spasms I try the lying-down exercise mentioned in the section on back pain. If that doesn't work within about fifteen minutes (it usually does), I take a muscle relaxant (see the list of pain medicines below). Then I get back on the floor for about twenty minutes, until the medicine starts to take effect. (It takes longer if I've just eaten.) The way I understand it, spasms cause pain and pain causes spasms. My goal is to break the pain-spasm cycle as quickly as I can.

I have also learned that headaches are very hard to get rid of if I don't take action promptly. With me, headaches are rarely bad enough to qualify as migraine, but they can hang on and on for weeks, even for months. I can't take aspirin, but if acetaminophen (Tylenol) works within an hour, that's the end of the headache. If not, I take an NSAID. I rarely need anything stronger, but I have a supply of prescription acetaminophen and codeine on hand for real emergencies.

The point is to start with the mildest pain preparation possible and work up only if you must. I think that people who try to be brave about pain that is worse than a background nuisance are doing themselves a real disservice.

A word about NSAIDs: Several kinds are available without prescriptions. In addition to reducing inflammation, which is not part of fibromyalgia, they have an analgesic (pain-relieving) effect. Aspirin is an NSAID; aside from its tendency to cause indigestion in some people—which can usually be avoided by drinking a glass of milk or eating something solid along with it—it has few side effects and is safe for most people. (Aspirin should *never* be given to a child without consulting the child's physician.) Other NSAIDs include ibuprofen (Advil, Motrin) and naproxen sodium (Aleve). Some people find that ibuprofen causes them to retain water. A moderate amount of water retention is probably not dangerous, but it can add to the discomfort you already feel. More potent doses of some NSAIDs are available by prescription, or your doctor may tell you to take more of the over-the-counter form than the package label suggests. Some drugstore analgesics contain caffeine—they may help with your pain, but they may also keep you awake at night. If you have a sleep problem, read the package contents.

If nothing you can buy without a prescription helps you, you may want to talk to your doctor about the drugs on this list.

• Cyclobenzaprine (Flexeril) is a muscle relaxant. It is probably the second most often prescribed drug for fibromyalgia. Some people find that it makes them drowsy, so try it at home the first time when you don't have to drive or operate machinery. If you get a dry mouth when taking Flexeril, keep water handy for sipping, or suck on sugarless hard candies. People with fibromyalgia usually take a 10-mg tablet one to three times per day. One study found that the higher dose does no better than the lower dose. If you're taking one a day, you'll probably get the most benefit by taking it about an hour before bedtime.

• Tramadol (Ultram) is a new analgesic in the United States, but it has been in use in Germany since 1977. According to the manufacturer's literature, the most frequently reported side effects are constipation, nausea, dizziness, headache, drowsiness, and vomiting. These side effects are about the same as those experienced by people taking acetaminophen (Tylenol with Codeine No. 3), but that is a narcotic drug and Ultram is not. Normal dose is one or two 50-mg tablets every four to six hours, with a maximum of eight tablets a day.

• Metaxalone (Skelaxin) is a sedative pain reliever. Although its name seems to suggest that it relaxes skeletal muscles (that is, all the muscles that attach to bones) that is not its direct effect, according to the manufacturer, who says its action in human beings has not been established but may be due to depression of the central nervous system. Adverse side effects may include nausea, vomiting, upset stomach, drowsiness, dizziness, headache, nervousness, and a slight rash, with or without itching. Recommended dose is two 400-mg tablets three or four times a day.

• Ketorolac (Toradol) is an injectable NSAID used to treat acute migraine. Injected into the muscle, a 30-mg dose usually relieves pain, nausea, and vomiting within an hour, with relief lasting up to six hours. A larger dose gives relief for a longer time, but it does not give more relief during the time it is effective. A 10-mg pill is also available. Toradol is usually reserved for people who have repeated migraines. Side effects may include nausea, constipation, diarrhea, dizziness, sleepiness, dry mouth, insomnia, nervousness, tremor, itching, and urinary retention. It is not recommended for use beyond five days at a time. People who are taking aspirin or heart or high blood pressure medications should not take Toradol.

• Sumatriptan (Imitrex) is another injectable form of migraine relief. It may alleviate the pain, nausea, and light sensitivity of migraine in as little as 20 minutes. It should not be given to people with heart, liver, or kidney problems. It is usually injected beneath the skin in a 6-mg dose. Two injections in twenty-four hours is the maximum dose.

• Propranolol (Inderal) one of a class of drugs known as beta-blockers, is normally used to reduce high blood pressure (hypertension), but it has been found to help prevent migraine. This class of drugs has complex interactions with other drugs, so be sure that the doctor who prescribes it knows everything else that you are taking, whether for pain or any other purpose.

Narcotic Drugs

The use of narcotics for fibromyalgia pain is highly controversial. Charged with preventing addiction and the illegal use of addictive drugs, the U.S. Drug Enforcement Agency pays close attention to doctors who prescribe narcotics and can make life quite miserable for those who do so liberally. Unfortunately, this agency fails to differentiate between people who seek narcotics for psychological or recreational reasons and those for whom narcotics offer the only real relief from physical pain. Indeed, most people who require narcotics for pain relief do not become addicted to them. Also state boards that regulate physicians can be hard on those they consider to be too liberal in prescribing controlled substances. Doctors, therefore, are apt to be cautious about prescribing narcotics, particularly for people who ask for them. Another deterrent is the fact that some of those rare individuals who have become addicted have successfully sued their doctors. One doctor told me, "I have had three patients who confessed that they were asking for increasingly higher doses of narcotics because they were selling them. If word gets out that one gives out narcotics liberally, one is soon deluged with the kind of drug-seeking patients that make it no fun to go to work each day."

The two most commonly prescribed narcotic drugs are acetaminophen (Tylenol with Codeine No. 3; there are lesser strengths numbered 1 and 2), and hydrocodone bitartrate (Vicodin), which also contains acetaminophen.

From the fibromyalgic's perspective, however, perhaps the

most important reason to avoid narcotics if possible is that they block deep sleep and can make fibromyalgia symptoms worse the next day. I have taken narcotic drugs for pain relief in my worst times, and the thing about them that bothered me most (aside from the druggy feeling, which I detest) was that they seem to shut my lower digestive tract down completely, giving new meaning to the word constipation. Lucky for me, my pain rarely gets so bad that I need narcotics.

Nonmedical Pain Management Techniques

In a way, I've been lucky with fibromyalgia. It started when I was a little girl and because my parents showed no concern about it, I grew up thinking that pain was normal. I learned to put my pain into the background and pay little attention to it. This worked—and still works—for me with pain I would describe as aching, dull, pulsating—constant pains that don't distract me from whatever I am doing. It does not work with sudden, sharp, stabbing, intermittent pains that demand my attention on an unpredictable schedule. I have another technique for dealing with that kind of pain. If I can't work because of pain, I simply give in to it. I let the pain take over, and eventually it becomes bearable.

When you feel pain, your automatic response is to tighten the muscles in the area that hurts, but tense muscles make the pain worse. To counteract this effect, if the pain is so bad that it's forcing me to concentrate on it—and after I've satisfied myself that it is caused by fibromyalgia and not a medical emergency—I lie down and let the pain take over. I concentrate on relaxing the tense muscles one by one, and on letting the pain flow freely through my body instead of trying to block it, which concentrates the pain in one place. I sometimes describe this as "making myself one with the pain." It works for me, and I think it can work for you.

Contrary to common sense, when you stop fighting pain, it doesn't get worse—its intensity decreases and it becomes more manageable. It may take as much as an hour to obtain relief, but I know from experience that I can go about my business sooner if I give in to the pain than if I don't. If my relaxation techniques don't make the pain go away entirely (about half the time this is true for me), then I take an analgesic when I get up. I think the single most important thing a person with fibromyalgia can learn is how to manage and minimize the pain that comes with FM, rather than fight it and make things worse.

When doctors examine a person who has fibromyalgia, they invariably find taut, tense muscles, often exacerbated by poor posture. Learning to stretch tight muscles properly brings great benefits to fibromyalgics. Stretching should be gentle and bilateral. Whatever you do on the right side you must do also on the left.

If you know that your posture is poor, perhaps you can get your doctor to refer you to a physical therapist for exercises to improve it. Poor posture yields cramped muscles and reduces the amount of oxygen available to the muscles and organs of your body. Think about standing up straight—not rigidly, but as though there were a plumb line from the top of your head to your feet, following your spine. If you balance your head on top of your spine, you will be less inclined to slouch and to compress your lungs. Be mindful of the relative position of your head and spine when you sit, too.

Massage and Physical Therapy

Many people who have fibromyalgia benefit from massage or physical therapy. For most people who have health insurance, physical therapy is a less expensive option—most insurers will pay for it if a doctor prescribes it—but it is not necessarily preferable. Physical therapists are usually trained to help people regain strength and flexibility in injured limbs by means of repetitive exercises, for example, bending and extending a knee or raising and lowering an arm. But repetitive motion exercises are usually not good for people with fibromyalgia. If you do ten repetitions of an exercise, you may feel all right that day, but the next day, or even two or three days later, you may feel extremely sore in the muscles that you exercised. There is a good reason for this, and it's one you should understand so that you can explain it to your physical therapist, if necessary.

As you read in Chapter 2, when muscles work they often develop microscopic tears. Growth hormone, secreted during deep sleep, fixes the tears. If you do not get sufficient restorative sleep, you do not secrete sufficient growth hormone and your muscles do not get repaired properly or promptly. Movement, particularly the kind that makes you stretch muscles and then contract them, is a form of vigorous exercise. Microtrauma, the tiny muscle tears, occur in anyone who exercises, whether or not they have fibromyalgia. But the tears in people without FM get repaired promptly. Also, if they do the same exercise for several days in a row, the muscle soreness disappears due to something known as the training effect—the muscles simply fail to report pain, and meanwhile they are being repaired. This is not true in people with fibromyalgia: The training effect does not take place, and muscle repair is delayed. That is why repetitive-motion exercises are not good for most people with fibromyalgia.

There is a saying, "If the only tool you have is a hammer, every problem looks like a nail." This is true not only of carpenters but also of all of us. The physical therapist who is taught to help people only by repetitive-motion exercise becomes convinced that repetitive-motion exercise will help every patient who has restricted motion and is in pain. Similarly, the orthopedic surgeon sees every problem as one that can be helped by surgery; the rheumatologist tends to think in terms of NSAIDs and steroids; the psychiatrist thinks that every problem has its basis in the psyche.

Just as physical therapists who don't understand how FM affects people can make you hurt more, so can massage therapists who know only one method of massage and think it is the answer to all ills. There are too many different schools and techniques of massage to discuss here. The best way to find a massage therapist is by word of mouth: Go to a local FM support group and ask people there for recommendations.

Sometimes massage is uncomfortable, but it should not be extremely painful, and the person who does the massage should stop immediately if you say it hurts too much—not more than you can bear, mind you, but more than you want to endure. A massage therapist who coaxes you to continue after you say to stop is not helping you. Your muscles are more apt to go into spasms, and at least they will be more tense after you are done. That only makes things worse. Massage can be wonderfully relaxing, but only if it is done by someone who understands fibromyalgia and who respects your knowledge of your own body.

Some people with fibromyalgia find relief using either a transcutaneous electrical nerve stimulation (TENS) machine or an alpha stim machine. A TENS unit stimulates the nerves electrically until they lose all sensation temporarily, giving relief from pain. Not everyone is helped, and some people think it makes the pain worse, but it may be worth discussing with your health care provider. In some cases, if a doctor prescribes it, insurance will cover either the rental or purchase of a TENS unit.

Alpha stim is a method of making your body relax. Your brain emits alpha waves when you are relaxed, in a meditative sort of state. One person with fibromyalgia told me, "Alpha stim changed my life. It gave me the first control over my pain that I've ever had." Alpha stim runs a very low frequency electrical current to a clip that you place on your earlobe. Rather than produce an electric shock that eliminates the nerve's ability to report pain, this method restores the electrical-chemical state that exists when a person is not in pain. It helps bring about relaxation, which reduces the level of pain, according to people who have had good results using it.

CASE HISTORY: DONALD, 41, UNIVERSITY PROFESSOR

Donald is the only one in his family with a fibromyalgia diagnosis, although he suspects his mother may have had it. "It is only now that I can appreciate all the aches and pains she had, and the fatigue that often sent her to bed," he says. Five years and seven physicians after his symptoms first appeared, he was diagnosed with both FM and CFS. The problem began with a flulike illness one autumn in the late 1980s. "I had several blood tests, none of which showed anything. The two doctors I saw were baffled," he reports. The illness recurred the following fall. Since then Donald has had constant aches and pains. His ears have become hypersensitive to the cold. "The slightest cool breeze gives me a terrible earache," he says. Two years ago the pain and fatigue intensified, again in the autumn. This time a new symptom appeared: orchitis, or inflammation of the testicles. This symptom waxes and wanes, but it is always present. Looking for diagnosis and relief, Donald saw three urologists and a neurologist, and finally went to a famous clinic, where he received the FM/CFS diagnosis.

Donald's other symptoms include "perpetual mental fog, forgetfulness, the inability to concentrate or express myself clearly, especially in speech," and problems with dizziness and lack of balance. His hips, thighs, and knees ache incessantly.

At night, Donald is troubled by restless leg syndrome, a condition in which the legs (and sometimes other parts of the body) are subject to involuntary motion and the feeling that the person must keep them moving, thus making it difficult to fall asleep. No pain is involved, but Donald says, "It drives me nuts."

Donald is a light sleeper. In the morning, he says, "My bed looks like a disaster area, with covers all over the place. When I get up in the morning . . . I ache all over and feel more tired than when I went to bed. It doesn't matter if I've slept five, seven, or nine hours—I always feel terrible in the morning."

His nonwork life is surprisingly vigorous: two rounds of golf a week, although he notes that his game has deteriorated greatly; table tennis one night a week ("We play a rough game," he remarks), and visiting friends or dining out on weekends. Asked how he keeps from overextending himself, Donald replies, "I don't, and that may be part of the problem."

Donald told his department head about his fibromyalgia just over a year ago, but thinks he may have forgotten. The department secretaries know that he hasn't been feeling well, but he hasn't shared any of the details. "I feel sorry for my students on days that my mind and body are having trouble and I'm only able to deliver 50 percent," he adds. Donald feels unable to cope as well as he used to with the thirty-five undergraduate and graduate students to whom he is faculty adviser, the laboratory projects he oversees, and the daily administrative routine of academic life. He bemoans the fact that "work has become work, and is no longer much fun."

Donald isn't getting much sympathy at home. "I suppose it's hard for anyone to sense what another feels like, if they have never had to deal with something like FM," he says. "My wife seems to think that it's all in my head and that it will go away someday. I try not to bother her or my daughter too much. I try to mask my depression and pain as well as possible." He continues to do the household vacuuming and all the yardwork without complaint, "but at a somewhat slower and less vigorous pace. Sometimes it's tough," he says.

His orchitis forced him to abstain from sex for a few months, but intimate relations are back in his life, although the testicular aches and pains remain.

Women with fibromyalgia outnumber men by about ten to one. But men are often more reluctant to ask for help with the tasks fibromyalgia makes difficult (running the vacuum cleaner is the one chore women mention most often as torturous) or to seek the emotional support that is sometimes all that makes the condition tolerable. Giving up golf and table tennis might impress his family with the severity of his aches and pains, but physical inactivity might well make his condition worse. There are no easy answers when fibromyalgia is the question.

CHAPTER FOUR

Illnesses Similar or Related to Fibromyalgia

THE characteristic of fibromyalgia that is most distressing to people who have it and most baffling to physicians is that many of its symptoms mimic other ailments. Too often, confronted with a set of symptoms that suggest the patient has disease X and a set of test results that say the patient doesn't have disease X, the doctor assumes that the patient is faking or imagining the symptoms and really isn't sick at all. Even the most sympathetic doctors must sometimes wonder about the patient who comes in with all kinds of symptoms, but whose tests say that nothing is wrong.

For patients, this situation is embarrassing and frustrating, sometimes frightening. It's easy to begin to doubt yourself when you feel terrible and the tests say you're fine. It's also dangerous. If you've seen your doctor six different times with six different complaints and been told that nothing is wrong with you, you may be tempted to ignore your symptoms the seventh time, when something entirely apart from FM is the problem, you really do need treatment, and a cure is indeed possible.

How can you tell the difference? Unfortunately, often you can't and you really should call your doctor, at least for a consultation by telephone. Gradually, however, you will probably develop an instinct about what is and what is not part of the fibromyalgia syndrome. Meanwhile, if you're not sure, make that call if the symptoms are such that you would call the doctor if you didn't have FM. You'll be safer that way.

This chapter describes some of the problems that often accompany fibromyalgia and suggests some ways that others have found to alleviate the symptoms. If you have a new set of symptoms that don't seem remotely life-threatening (this excludes symptoms such as chest pain and shortness of breath), you might try some of these suggestions for a day or two before seeking medical help. But use good judgment: If your instincts tell you to call the doctor, by all means do so.

Also in this chapter are descriptions of other conditions sometimes associated with fibromyalgia. The purpose of including them is to help you understand where FM fits in the scheme of things, and to remind you that you may have fibromyalgia *and* something else at the same time.

Irritable Bowel Syndrome

One of the most upsetting problems associated with fibromyalgia is a gastrointestinal disturbance known as irritable bowel syndrome (IBS), which one person with fibromyalgia termed "the cry of the wild gut." IBS involves painful, crampy diarrhea, sometimes so severe that people who have it must plan their days around the need for several urgent trips to the bathroom (IBS is usually, though not always, worse in the morning). Alternating with diarrhea may be extended bouts of constipation. Indeed, this may be your tip-off that you have IBS and not colitis or Crohn's disease, which are characterized by chronic diarrhea alone. But you may not be able to wait to see if constipation follows an attack of diarrhea; prolonged diarrhea can lead to dehydration and severe mineral deficiencies, which can by themselves be life-threatening. Gastrointestinal viruses and indigestion from spoiled food rarely last more than three days, so you might want to make that your rule of thumb when deciding whether to check with the doctor.

If Crohn's disease and colitis are ruled out, you may also want to consider the possibility that food sensitivities are causing the problem. Lactose (milk sugar) intolerance is a common cause of diarrhea. You can screen for it yourself, by eliminating all dairy products from your diet for a couple of weeks. If your symptoms disappear, there are preparations that you can take to provide the enzyme whose absence causes the problem.

Having eliminated all other possibilities, the best approach to IBS is to pay attention to your diet. Here is another place where common sense works against you: It is reasonable to assume that since leafy green vegetables provide the roughage needed to make our bowels move, then the cure for diarrhea is to avoid them. Nothing could be farther from the truth. Plenty of fiber, possibly including an over-the-counter fiber preparation from your pharmacy's laxative section, is the best defense against IBS. In addition, many people discover that their IBS improves dramatically when they cut out refined sugars (be warned that some fiber preparations contain sugar; avoid them). Caffeine and alcohol are two other irritants that should be avoided while your intestines are acting up. Over-the-counter antidiarrheal medications can help some; there are also prescription drugs to calm your gut, but these are not a long-term solution. Another over-the-counter drug that helps some people, although no one knows why, is diphenhydramine (Benadryl), which is an antihistamine used to treat allergies. One or two 25-mg capsules may bring prompt relief.

If your IBS swings back the other way, making you constipated, try increasing your fiber intake and drink plenty of water (eight, eight-ounce glasses of water a day is not overdoing it, especially in hot weather or when you are exerting yourself physically). If that doesn't work, try a mild laxative, possibly one that contains a stool softener. Do not take a laxative that contains a bowel stimulant; you're likely to find yourself bouncing between diarrhea and constipation with great frequency.

Irritable Bladder (Urethral Syndrome)

If you have ever had a urinary tract infection (UTI) you are not likely to forget the experience—frequent, urgent, burning, painful urination. In fibromyalgia, however, many people experience what seems like a UTI caused by bacteria in the bladder or urethra (urinary tube), except that no bacteria are found when the urine is analyzed under a microscope (normally, urine is sterile—that is, it doesn't have germs in it). This is irritable bladder syndrome, sometimes called female urethral syndrome. Men are less susceptible because their urethras are longer and less likely to become irritated. Because the letters *IBS* already describe irritable bowel syndrome (above), we'll call the irritable bladder condition urethral syndrome, or US.

This is one of those times when it's hard to know whether to call the doctor or wait for the symptoms to go away. If you go to the doctor, you will probably be given an antibiotic and a pain reliever that works specifically in the urinary tract. If you do nothing, the problem will probably resolve itself within a few days, so there's not much risk in trying to handle it yourself before seeing the doctor. There are some situations, however, in which you should call the doctor immediately.

- If your urine has a foul odor
- If you see blood in your urine
- If you are running a fever

These may be signs of a more serious infection that can be cured only with medication.

If you try to handle things yourself, there are two things you can do, and you should do both. First, spend some time sitting in the bathtub in water that is hot, but not so hot as to be uncomfortable. Sitz baths, as they are called, give rapid though temporary relief and can be repeated as often as convenient. Second, get some cranberry pills or capsules and take one each time you urinate. Keep taking them for a few days after the pain or burning is gone. Drinking cranberry juice is a time-honored remedy for US. It works for most people, but I recommend cranberry pills instead because the juice is usually full of sweeteners that may trigger other problems. If bacteria are present, the sugars in cranberry juice may well feed the germs and make things worse; they may also cause an overgrowth of yeast or symptoms of hypoglycemia. If you can't find cranberry pills or capsules (most health food stores carry them), vitamin C is an adequate substitute. Take one 500-mg pill or more, if you can tolerate it, each time you urinate.

It's hard to accept the need for this, but if you are plagued by US, whether or not you're having your doctor treat you for it, buy a box of incontinent pads—and wear them. You'll have more peace of mind, and you may well save your dignity, too.

If you are experiencing FM-caused urinary urgency, the best course of action is to avoid caffeine and alcohol altogether. You may find that eliminating caffeine—also present in tea, chocolate, and cola drinks—is all it takes to cure your irritable bladder.

Both irritable bowel and irritable bladder problems are sometimes caused by myofascial trigger points in the abdomen. Information on myofascial pain syndrome and trigger points appears in chapter 5.

Circulatory Problems

Poor peripheral circulation—cold feet and hands, possibly accompanied by numbness—is another vexing problem familiar to many people who have fibromyalgia. A more extreme condition is known as Raynaud's disease or Raynaud's phenomenon. Generally, the term Raynaud's disease is used when there appears to be no underlying cause, whereas the same problem is called Raynaud's phenomenon when it is a secondary characteristic to another disorder, such as FM. True Raynaud's disease is uncommon. We'll use the term Raynaud's here to describe both forms, since they affect people in essentially the same way.

Raynaud's is characterized by spasms of the small blood vessels in the hands and feet. The affected area may turn red, white, or blue, or all three; the sensation is one of extreme cold, both to the person who has the disorder and to anyone who touches the person's hands or feet. The fingers and toes may turn numb; they may also ache, burn, or tingle.

The cause of Raynaud's is not known; there is some evidence to suggest that it runs in families. Early episodes may involve only one or two fingertips. Attacks may be triggered by exposure to cold or by emotional upset. Though it is uncomfortable, Raynaud's does not often cause any harm. Attacks may last for minutes or hours, but are rarely severe enough to cause tissue loss. In rare cases, tiny, painful ulcers may appear on the fingertips.

Raynaud's is rarely severe enough to warrant taking drugs to cure it, but if it's troubling you, it's worth mentioning to your physician.

There are several things you can do to avoid episodes of Raynaud's. First, dress warmly. Dress in layers, even in summer, so that you can take things off and put them on as your internal temperature dictates. When the weather is cold, remember that you lose a large percentage of body heat from your head, so wear a hat. Buy your winter shoes big and wear two pairs of socks. Wear gloves. Keep as warm as you can. Warm—*not hot*—water soaks help greatly to relieve painful cold hands and feet. If you smoke tobacco, stop. Nicotine has been shown time and again to constrict blood vessels, decreasing the availability of oxygen to the extremities. Aerobic exercise is your third line of defense. It stimulates circulation, which is what you need most.

Cognitive Problems

Aside from pain, probably the most vexing aspect of FM is the effect it can have on your cognitive abilities—to remember things, figure out problems, come up with the right words or names, and just plain think. Some people feel that they are in a fog much of the time. They have trouble concentrating on what people are saying. They have difficulty remembering where they have put things—even if they just put it down a couple minutes ago—are unable to remember what they just read, forget things they've promised to do, and miss appointments.

These symptoms usually come and go; they are most likely to be worse when your other FM symptoms are worse. I find that when I'm sleeping well and my pain is under control, I rarely have these problems. The inability to concentrate and think clearly is a symptom of depression, and some physicians assume that is the case when fibromyalgics complain of it, but there is ample evidence that these cognitive difficulties have a physical cause apart from depression. Some doctors think an abnormality in a portion of the brain is to blame. Others say our brains don't get enough oxygen, which causes them to malfunction. It's important that you understand this: The cognitive problems that accompany FM have nothing to do with Alzheimer's disease, nor do they have anything to do with brain damage. Some of the medications people take for fibromyalgia actually cause these symptoms as a side effect, so as the rest of your FM gets better, the brain dysfunction problems may get worse. If this is the case, adjusting or changing the medication may provide the answer.

Fortunately, there are things you can do to compensate for fibromyalgia's "brain fog." As is true with every other aspect of learning to live well with FM, you'll have to experiment to find out what works best for you. Here are some suggestions.

• Be methodical. The saying "A place for everything and everything in its place" should be the fibromyalgic's slogan. I keep my car keys on a sliding hook that I clip to a ring on my handbag every time I get out of the car, even to come into my own house. My sunglasses are in my handbag at all times, unless I am wearing them. By being methodical in this manner, I always know where my glasses and car keys are.

• Make lists. I couldn't imagine going to the supermarket without a shopping list; I'd surely forget half of what I need to buy. If I have several errands to run, I list them all in the order in which I intend to do them, then check each one off as it is completed.

• Take notes. I keep a spiral notebook and a pencil next to the telephone. Before I answer the phone I pick up the pencil, so I am ready to write down the name of the person who is calling as soon as it's said. If I make an appointment or agree to do something as a result of the call, I write that in the book, too.

• **Make it difficult to forget.** I put reminder notes to myself in places I can't miss them—on the bathroom mirror, on my computer monitor, on my desk chair, on my pillow. As much as possible, when I think of doing something, I try to do it immediately. I learned this from a successful man I once interviewed for a magazine article. I don't think he had FM, but he said he had so many things on his mind that he simply had to do things the minute he thought of them or he'd probably forget to do them entirely.

• **Establish routines.** Being organized and methodical does not come naturally to me, but I have discovered that if I do something the same way, day after day, for about three weeks, the habit is established and I no longer have to think about it—I just do it.

People who like to try nutritional supplements for FM problems may want to try ginkgo (*Ginkgo biloba*) capsules or the amino acid L-glutamine. If "brain fog" is a serious problem for you, you might want to mention this to your physician.

Ear and Hearing Problems

For people who have fibromyalgia, ear problems fall into two categories: vertigo and hearing loss.

Vertigo is the feeling that everything around you is in motion when you know it's not. It differs from dizziness, in which you feel that you are in motion, usually spinning or wobbling. Some of the medications commonly used for FM can cause vertigo; if this happens to you, tell your physician immediately. In addition to being uncomfortable, vertigo is a dangerous condition if you have to drive a car or operate machinery. A change in the dosage may be all that is required to set you straight.

About one-third of people with FM have tinnitus, continual noise in the ears. It may be a buzz, ring, roar, whistle, or hiss, or it may be a combination of these, varying over time. Tinnitus can have many causes, the easiest to fix being impacted wax in the ear. There is no specific medical or surgical cure for tinnitus. Many people who have it found they can get to sleep more easily if they play soft music to mask the noise.

Tinnitus is most often accompanied by some degree of hearing loss. In some cases, the hearing loss comes and goes and is accompanied by a feeling of pressure in the affected ear, but a doctor looking in the ear can see no cause for the pressure. Gradually, over a few days or weeks, hearing returns to normal. Fortunately, it rarely attacks both ears at once.

Hypoglycemia

Hypoglycemia, which means low blood sugar, is a common complaint among people who have fibromyalgia. Strictly speaking, their blood sugar is not low all the time, as would be true with real hypoglycemia, but it drops so low and so suddenly at times that the symptoms are similar to those of the real thing.

The symptoms of hypoglycemia are many and varied: headache, usually in the forehead or the top of the head, dizziness, irritability, fatigue, depression, nervousness, difficulty with memory and concentration, heart palpitations or pounding, trembling hands, cold sweats, a feeling of impending doom, leg cramps, numbness or tingling of the hands and/or feet, flushing, panic attacks, and sometimes fainting.

If you think you have hypoglycemia, your doctor may order a fasting blood sugar or glucose tolerance test. For both tests, you appear at the laboratory first thing in the morning, without having had anything to eat or drink since the previous evening. For a fasting blood sugar test, the technician draws one vial of blood and tests it to see what your blood sugar level is when you haven't had anything to eat for about twelve hours. The average fasting blood sugar is 100; rates of 85 to 115 are usually considered within normal limits. If your fasting blood sugar is too high, it means that you have diabetes. If it is too low, you have real hypoglycemia. If you think you have hypoglycemia and you have FM, your fasting blood sugar will probably be within normal range—until you have something to eat.

That's where the glucose tolerance test comes in. Glucose is a form of sugar. The test is designed to see how you handle sugar. Again, you go to the lab with an empty stomach. This time the technician draws some blood to get your fasting level; then you are instructed to drink a liquid containing a measured amount of glucose. It's sweet, for sure; how sweet it tastes depends on how much sugar you are accustomed to eating. The less sugar you normally eat, the sweeter things taste.

After you have had your glucose cocktail, you will probably be asked to sit in the waiting room awhile. The technician will draw blood from time to time; how often and how long will depend on the length of the test the doctor ordered. The report to the doctor will list your blood sugar levels each time blood was drawn. The longer the test continues, the more information the report will contain. If the test is done for too short a time, it will reveal little, if anything, of value. Therefore, if you have FM and think you have hypoglycemia, your doctor should order a five- or six-hour glucose tolerance test.

Here, in a nutshell, is what happens when you drink that glucose cocktail, or eat or drink anything that is loaded with sugar. Your pancreas, noting that your blood sugar level has risen, secretes insulin to digest the sugar and bring your blood sugar down to its normal level. (In diabetics, the pancreas fails to perform this job, necessitating insulin replacement.) If the blood sugar level drops too low, the adrenal glands secrete adrenaline, causing the liver to release part of its store of glycogen, which turns into glucose and brings the blood sugar level back up.

What seems to happen in fibromyalgics who have hypoglycemia symptoms is that the adrenal glands overreact, releasing adrenaline before the blood sugar level has dropped too low.

Adrenaline, the "fight-or-flight" hormone, is what you need to deal with an emergency; it gives you extra strength if you have to run or fight. But it also makes your breath come in short gasps, it makes your heart pound, and it makes you break out in a sweat. It's quite likely that panic attacks are really a reaction to a blood sugar level your adrenals think is too low.

The important information that a glucose tolerance test can reveal is not how soon your blood sugar level drops, but how far it drops when it does. That's why a long test is important if you think you have hypoglycemia. Your blood sugar level will rise quite rapidly after you drink the glucose, but it may not drop until well into the third or fourth hour. You'll know when it drops—you'll get the symptoms that you mentioned to the doctor. But if you have a three-hour test and the drop hits in the fourth hour, you've wasted your time and money, and the doctor won't get an accurate picture of what is happening. Table 4–1 shows the blood sugar levels of a hypoglycemic woman in a five-hour glucose tolerance test.

Hypoglycemia is diagnosed when the blood sugar goes more than 20 percent below the fasting blood sugar and is accompanied by symptoms. In this case, 20 percent below the fasting level would have been 74. This woman's blood sugar dropped at four hours to approximately 40 percent below the fasting level. At that point, she had a headache, broke out into a cold sweat,

HOUR	LEVEL	NORMAL RANGE
Fasting	93	85–115
½	158	120–170
1	142	120–170
2	148	70–120
3	100	85–115
4	57	85–115
5	61	85–115

Table 4-1: RESULTS OF A FIVE-HOUR GLUCOSE TOLERANCE TEST

had the chills and uncontrollable shaking, and felt that she was nearly in a stupor.

There is a vast difference in the effect of different kinds of sugars on your bloodstream. Sugar is a carbohydrate. So are bread, pasta, carrots, and apples. Carbohydrates are the mainstay of most people's diets, but sugar is a simple carbohydrate and the rest of the listed items are complex carbohydrates. Sugar is a simple carbohydrate because it has been refined, that is, everything that is not sugar (such as the B vitamins in sugarcane) has been stripped away. The same is true of white flour. Alcoholic beverages are simple sugars, too.

Complex carbohydrates have to be digested in your stomach before they get into your bloodstream. Simple carbohydrates— white sugar, white flour, and alcohol—go straight into your bloodstream without being digested. The impact on your blood sugar level is almost immediate, and the overreaction of your adrenal glands is almost a sure thing.

I wish I could tell you that you can cure your hypoglycemic symptoms immediately if you will give up simple sugars, but it's not that easy. Still, I urge you to do just that—stop eating simple carbohydrates. You will not get over your hypoglycemia if you don't. You may also need to eat several small meals each day instead of three big ones, to keep your blood sugar level stable while your adrenals relearn their job. You may have to give up many complex sugars temporarily, too. Fruit juices can trigger hypoglycemic episodes in some people, as can foods containing high-fructose corn syrup, other sweetening syrups, honey, and so forth. You'll probably have to give up pasta for a while—at least pasta made with wheat flour. When I was going through this, I discovered a kind of pasta made from ground-up Jerusalem artichokes. You can find artichoke pasta in any health food store and in many larger supermarkets. I doubt you could tell artichoke pasta from wheat pasta by look or by taste, but the difference in glucose reaction is noticeable.

If you give up all simple and most complex carbohydrates for a month or two, you can then safely begin to add foods back into your diet, starting with the least sweet and most complex. Do it gradually. Don't add more than one class of food at a time and wait a few days before adding anything else. You will quickly learn what does and does not agree with you and your adrenals, and you'll come to a place where you are happy with your diet and your diet is happy with you. But you can never add those simple carbohydrates back in, unless you want to go through this whole process all over again. Nondairy coffee creamers are another villain in the hypoglycemic's life. Actually, the caffeine in coffee and cola drinks has a similar effect on your blood sugar as granulated sugar, so you should avoid them, too.

It all sounds really grim, I know, but it need not be so bad. Yes, you're going to have to read the labels on food packages for the rest of your life. You'll be amazed at the things manufacturers put sugar in. But as you give up sugar, everything else tastes sweeter. And you'll find that your cravings for sugar eventually go away. The pectin in apples is good for stabilizing blood sugar, so you may want to put apples back into your diet as one of the first carbohydrates you try. Nuts, particularly almonds and walnuts, are good snacks for hypoglycemics. Cashews are full of natural sugars and should be avoided until you've added back in almost all other complex carbohydrates. When you start eating bread again, make it dark, whole-grain breads. Avoid white bread and white flour in any form, as much as you can.

While you are gathering your courage to get over your hypoglycemia, keep in mind that fats are good for stabilizing blood sugar. If you have a hypoglycemic attack, assuming you can tolerate milk, a glass of 2 percent or whole (4 percent) milk will help you quickly. Peanut butter on a preferably whole-wheat cracker is also a good emergency aid.

There is a drug to combat hypoglycemia that has recently come on the market, but its side effects include nausea and loss of appetite. Frankly, I think you'd have to be a serious sugar addict to take a pill that makes you feel nauseated just so you can go on eating sugar. Some people find help in regulating their blood sugar by taking chromium picolinate, a tablet you can find in a health food store. If you try this, be sure to follow the label instructions to know how much to take, and do not exceed the recommended amount. Chromium is a heavy metal; you need only a tiny bit of it in your body. And you must not think that chromium picolinate will allow you to eat sugar. You can't, unless you are willing to accept a life of panic attacks and all those other symptoms.

Mitral Valve Prolapse

The mitral valve is one of the four valves that open and close to move blood through the heart. Mitral valve prolapse (MVP), which sounds at lot more dangerous than it is, occurs when the mitral valve bulges upward during a heartbeat. The valve, whose job it is to move blood from one chamber in the heart to another, can't get a good seal. Thus, it allows a small quantity of blood to seep backward into the next chamber. Mitral valve prolapse occurs in roughly 75 percent of people who have fibromyalgia. A comparably high percentage of people who are diagnosed first with MVP are later found to have FM.

MVP does not cause chest pain. In fact, ordinarily the only symptom of MVP is a heart murmur, a sound that occurs when the valve closes. Doctors may hear it when they use a stethoscope to listen to your heart. Both FM and MVP are associated with headaches, fatigue, and irritable bowel syndrome. The connection between the two is not known. MVP involves a change in the connective tissue of the heart, but there are no other known connective tissue changes in fibromyalgia. Some doctors who suspect MVP will want you to have an echocardiogram, an ultrasound examination of the heart, but whether the echocardiogram will show the prolapse depends on what kind of fibromyalgia day you are having.

MVP is of little importance, unless you have other cardiac problems. As an added precaution, however, many physicians prescribe a course of antibiotics for people who have it before they undergo any dental work (including cleaning) or surgery. The idea is to prevent bacteria from entering the heart and causing infection there. People who don't want to, or can't take antibiotics might want to consider taking extra vitamin C, a natural antibiotic, in the same situations. Doctors generally tell people with MVP to avoid sugar and caffeine, increase fluids, and engage in moderate exercise—the same things you should be doing to alleviate symptoms of fibromyalgia.

Premenstrual Syndrome

If you have FM and have menstrual periods, you probably do have premenstrual syndrome (PMS). Most of the symptoms of PMS are just like those of FM, only worse: headache, insomnia, back pain, abdominal cramps, mental confusion, and emotional upset. As anyone who has ever experienced it can tell you, PMS is terrible. It can keep you home and in bed, it can make you a nervous wreck, it can make you a screaming shrew, or it can cause you to cry uncontrollably. FM accentuates these symptoms.

B-complex vitamins, calcium and magnesium, and over-the-counter pain-relieving medicines help to some extent. Doctors sometimes prescribe hormones for women with extremely bad PMS. Serotonin seems to be at its lowest at PMS time, which is why premenstrual women so often crave carbohydrates, especially chocolate. As in other situations, sugar may help for a short time, but it makes things worse in the long run, increasing the tendency toward insomnia and anxiety attacks. Whereas every bone in your body may want to be in bed when you have PMS, walking is often one of the best things you can do to relieve it.

Reflux

Esophageal reflux is a condition in which the contents of the stomach exert back pressure on the muscular valve between the stomach and the bottom of the esophagus, forcing liquefied, partially digested food and stomach acid back into the esophagus. It is sometimes referred to as heartburn or acid indigestion. Reflux is a problem for many people who have fibromyalgia.

Over-the-counter antacids may help. In severe cases, doctors sometimes recommend cimetidine (Tagamet) or ranitidine (Zantac), two powerful antacids. If you are in the habit of eating until your stomach feels full, you may find that stopping before you get the full sensation is all it takes to avoid reflux. At any rate, it's certainly worth a try.

Reflux can also occur during sleep. Some people find relief by propping the head of their bed up on cinder blocks or sleeping on a wedge-shaped pillow that elevates the upper part of the body. Reflux can also be caused by obstructive sleep apnea (Chapter 2).

Hypothyroidism

Because the classic symptoms of an underactive thyroid gland so closely mimic those of fibromyalgia—muscle pain, weakness, morning stiffness, fatigue, water retention, constipation, Raynaud's phenomenon, cognitive problems, loss of libido, and depression—your doctor should test your thyroid function before deciding that FM is your problem, or your only problem. Many people with fibromyalgia also have underactive thyroids. Treatment with thyroid replacement hormone should relieve the symptoms within a few weeks, if hypothyroidism is the only problem. Eating foods rich in iodine (especially seafood) helps strengthen the thyroid gland.

Chronic Fatigue Syndrome

There is considerable disagreement as to whether fibromyalgia and chronic fatigue syndrome (CFS, also known as chronic fatigue and immune deficiency syndrome, or CFIDS) are the same disorder with different names. The argument in favor of their being the same is that the two syndromes have many of the same signs and symptoms. Some people say that whether you are diagnosed with FM or CFS depends on whether your doctor is a rheumatologist or an internist, or whether your primary complaint is pain or fatigue.

Each syndrome has a set of diagnostic criteria. For FM, the criteria were established by the American College of Rheumatology and include chronic pain lasting more than three months; pain in all four quadrants of the body, including the spine; and painful tenderness in at least eleven of eighteen specific locations (see chapter 1, figure 1). The criteria for CFS were established by a joint committee including members of the U.S. Centers for Disease Control and Prevention (CDC) and the National Institutes of Health (NIH). These criteria, which are more extensive than those for FM, are listed in table 4–2.

Using these criteria, you can form your own opinion as to whether FM and CFS are the same, and whether you have neither, one, or both. One thing that seems clear is that FM and CFS share certain common characteristics, but whereas there is evidence of neurohormonal dysfunction in each, the immune system seems to be compromised far more in CFS than in FM, where many people report that aside from having fibromyalgia, they seem to be more healthy than most people, and far less susceptible to colds and other contagious diseases.

Lyme Disease

If you have enough symptoms to make you think you have fibromyalgia, but not enough to qualify for a formal diagnosis (for example, not enough tender points, pain not sufficiently widespread or not having lasted long enough), ask your doctor to check you for Lyme disease. This is especially important if you have been in the woods recently.

Lyme disease is a bacterial infection that comes from being bitten by an infected tick. The tick may be gone, and there may be no signs of a bite, although if you notice it early enough you will see a red rash in a small circle, usually with a bull's-eye in

---

Table 4–2: CASE DEFINITION FOR THE CHRONIC FATIGUE
SYNDROME, DECEMBER 1994*

1. Clinically evaluated, unexplained persistent or re-
   lapsing chronic fatigue that is of new or definite
   onset (i.e., not lifelong), is not the result of ongoing exertion, is not substantially alleviated by rest,
   and results in substantial reduction in previous levels of occupational, educational, social, or personal
   activities.

2. The concurrent occurrence of four or more of the
   following symptoms: substantial impairment in
   short-term memory or concentration; sore throat;
   tender lymph nodes; muscle pain; multijoint pain
   without joint swelling or redness; headaches of a
   new type, pattern, or severity; nonrefreshing sleep;
   and postexertional malaise lasting more than
   twenty-four hours. These symptoms must have
   persisted or recurred during six or more consecutive months of illness and must not have predated
   the fatigue.

*Source: Centers for Disease Control

---

the middle. Many symptoms of Lyme disease mimic those of
fibromyalgia. There is a test for Lyme disease, but it's not very
accurate. False negatives (a result that says you don't have it
when you actually do) occur about 30 percent of the time; false
positives occur in only about 10 percent of cases.

Caught early enough, Lyme disease is cured in most cases by
a two-week course of the antibiotic doxycycline. Most people
diagnosed with chronic Lyme disease actually have FM, triggered by Lyme disease. It should not come as a great surprise
that sleep disturbance caused by Lyme disease could be the
triggering mechanism that brings on fibromyalgia in susceptible

people, but it would be a gross error to say that every case of FM is really a case of Lyme disease, or that Lyme disease causes FM.

Gulf War Syndrome

About 10,000 veterans of the Persian Gulf War have developed a set of familiar-sounding symptoms, including

- Recurring severe headaches
- Fatigue
- Joint and muscle pain (particularly in knees, ankles, shoulders, and back)
- Memory loss (often described as an inability to concentrate)
- Depression, irritability
- Insomnia
- Urinary urgency and frequency
- Diarrhea (sometimes bloody) or constipation
- Shortness of breath
- Chest pains
- Menstrual irregularities and pelvic pain in female veterans

When first reports of this syndrome, labeled by the press as Gulf War syndrome (GWS), first appeared, people who have fibromyalgia took notice with great interest. As this book was being written, the U.S. government released a report stating that there is no such thing as Gulf War syndrome. Coincidentally, the number of Gulf War veterans who have this collection of symptoms represents roughly 4 percent of those who served in the Gulf, just as people with fibromyalgia represent 4 percent of the population as a whole. It might be that the Gulf War was the triggering factor that turned these veterans into fibromyalgics. If you are, or know, one of these sufferers, treating the conditions as though it were FM might result in considerable improvement.

Postpolio Syndrome

Fibromyalgia occurs frequently in people who suffer from post-polio syndrome (PPS). Indeed, it may be that some of the symptoms of PPS *are* fibromyalgia, or that postpolio syndrome is one more trigger for FM. The virus that causes polio kills a certain percentage of the motor neurons that carry messages from the spinal cord to the muscles. The remaining neurons then take over the chore of bearing messages to the muscle fibers that were served by the killed neurons, giving each much more work to do than before the onset of polio. This is believed to make the neurons die early, causing the progressive weakness that characterizes postpolio syndrome, long after the virus is gone.

To the extent that postpolio symptoms are also symptoms of fibromyalgia, the person with PPS can be made to feel better by being treated for FM. Unfortunately, the muscle weakness is as yet untreatable.

CASE HISTORY: LIZ, 20, STUDENT

Liz was fourteen when a rheumatologist at a children's hospital diagnosed her fibromyalgia. She had been having migraine headaches from the age of five, and started being hypersensitive to light and noise at six. She went to her family doctor complaining of joint pain. He suspected that she had lupus, and sent her to the rheumatologist to have the diagnosis confirmed. "The rheumatologist poked at my tender points and said, 'You don't have lupus, you have fibrositis,'" Liz says. "My mom started crying because I didn't have lupus. I started crying because I had something with a weird name.

"I carry most of my tension in my neck and shoulders," she says. "I get both tension and migraine headaches. There have been times when I can barely move my neck without serious pain." Other symptoms include pain in her arms and hands and very dry skin ("painfully so during the winter, when showering hurts my skin"). Liz has had several episodes of serious but un-explained back pain. She takes care not to sit too long in one position, and finds relief in sleeping with her legs propped up on a pillow. "Occasionally I have chest pains that seem like a heart attack, but this is infrequent," she says.

Liz's most troublesome FM problem is irritable bowel syn-drome (IBS), with its alternating constipation and crampy diar-rhea. She also has an irritable bladder at times, which feels like a urinary tract infection and causes her to run to the bathroom even though her bladder is not full. Her menstrual periods are painful, and she cannot remain standing for long without severe pain in her legs and feet.

Liz is allergic to dust, ragweed, cats, grass, and tree pollens. Like most people with fibromyalgia, she cannot sleep without medication. "On my own, I am a very light sleeper and always have been. I awaken very easily," she says, and adds, "If I go off my sleeping medicine, the FM comes back with a vengeance." Liz lives in a college dormitory year-round. "I find that without medication to help me sleep, the noise of the other residents keeps me awake. I wish I didn't have to take meds, but I have little choice," she says.

Many people with fibromyalgia are reluctant to tell friends and associates about their condition. Liz is selective, but does not hesitate to tell people whom she thinks should know, usu-ally because it will help them to understand her needs. When she is feeling unsteady on her feet, Liz walks with a cane—not the ordinary drugstore variety, but one that is brightly decorated and, she says, "spiffy. It helps," she adds, "because often people notice the cane and not the fact that I need one. I find that people can be more understanding and considerate when I have the cane, and that bothers me. I don't like being singled out, but I am not too modest to use it."

Fortunately, Liz has a family that is "incredibly supportive. The only person who gets annoyed when I can't do things is my younger brother. He makes mean comments about my being lazy, but he gets annoyed with everyone, so I have learned to ignore his insults. I also don't go home very often, so this is usually not a problem," she says.

Many people find it difficult to maintain a social life when their FM is active, but Liz considers herself fortunate in this respect. "I have never enjoyed going to bars or dancing, so I don't feel that I am missing out on anything," she says. She spends eight to ten hours each week in a theater group, acting and directing, and centers her social life around the other members of the group, going to shows and out for coffee with them. She has also served on at least ten university committees. In addition, Liz works part time in a library, bookstore, and as an usher in a theater.

Learning to avoid agreeing to do more than she can handle comfortably is an ongoing problem for Liz. "I'm learning to say no and not feel guilty, but it's hard," she says. "Recently I had a bout of profound fatigue, not the usual tiredness that I've always lived with. I found that I had to break a few engagements, but I was honest and people understood. I am very aware of who in my life believes me and who does not, and this helps in deciding how to deal with someone."

Unlike many people who have fibromyalgia, Liz has told all three of her employers about her problems with fibromyalgia. "They are all very supportive, and I know how lucky I am. I have also never had to miss a shift because of FM, and that really helps," she says. Her co-workers know of her limitations, too, and willingly take on her share of the heavy lifting.

It's hard to take a positive approach to a life full of pain, but Liz has done so with considerable success. Her decorated cane tells people that she doesn't feel sorry for herself, making it easier for them to make allowances for the few limitations to which she admits. Although fibromyalgia is not a progressive condition—that is, it does not get worse as time passes—Liz has the stamina that comes with youth. As she grows older, she may feel the need to reduce what sounds like a frenetic schedule.

CHAPTER FIVE

Myofascial Pain Syndrome

I F you have ever looked carefully at a piece of red meat—a leg of lamb, for example—then you have a good idea of what your own muscles look like: long bands of fiber running parallel to each other, held in place by thin strips of connective tissue. The bits of muscle fiber are called myofibrils; *fascia* is another word for connective tissue. Myofascial pain, therefore, means pain coming from the muscle fiber and connective tissue.

The relationship between fibromyalgia and myofascial pain syndrome (MPS) remains unclear. Some researchers think that fibromyalgia leads to MPS; others think that MPS leads to FM. Still others think they are the same condition, and some think there is no relationship at all. In one study, investigators found signs of MPS in 68 percent of people with FM.[4]

Generally speaking, FM causes aches whereas MPS causes pain. The cognitive difficulties so many people who have fibromyalgia suffer from, the feeling upon arising of having been run over by a truck, the flulike aches, the lack of stamina, and the general sleep dysfunction that may cause these feelings—and certainly makes them worse—are fibromyalgia. Myofascial pain should be suspected as the cause of most of the rest of our symptoms. FM and MPS are treated differently.

MPS can masquerade as temporomandibular joint disorder (TMJ), migraine and tension headaches, carpal tunnel syndrome (CTS), thoracic outlet syndrome (TOS), appendicitis, sciatica, tennis elbow, bursitis, irritable bowel syndrome (IBS), and many other painful and debilitating conditions.[5]

If you suffer from one of these troublesome conditions, it is important that you and your physician consider that MPS is to blame, particularly before you agree to surgery to correct it. (See Appendix A for information on how to obtain a paper that lists these and other ailments that may be caused by MPS, as well as suggestions on how to treat them. No doctor can possibly know of every relevant article that appears in print, and yours might well appreciate receiving a copy of this paper from you.)

There are clear differences between FM and MPS. Fibromyalgia is characterized (among other things) by *widespread, generalized* aching. MPS is *localized;* that is, it causes pain in a specific area, which is not to say that there can only be one area of myofascial pain per person, but only that affected areas can be more readily defined. *Tender* points (TPs) are characteristic of fibromyalgia; they appear in predictable locations in muscles, over bones, or in the case of the knee, over fat. They are exquisitely sore when they are pressed. *Trigger* points (TrPs) are characteristic of MPS; they are found only in muscles. Pressing on a TrP will cause pain in some part of the body, but not necessarily at the site of the TrP. Indeed, one of the diagnostic criteria for TrPs is that the doctor can cause the pain of which the patient is complaining, simply by pressing on the trigger point. The TrP will be found as part of a taut band of muscle, which will twitch if the doctor touches it or inserts a needle into it.

The most important distinction is that whereas the tender points of FM may be more or less painful at any given time, they do not go away and are with us always. However, there are ways that may make the trigger points of MPS disappear. Whether they stay away forever depends on several factors, including how long they have existed, how they came to be in the first place, and how well the person who has them succeeds in avoiding the kinds of stimuli that caused them.

Investigators have identified several mechanisms that may lead to the formation of TrPs. Among them is injury to the muscle (macrotrauma) or to individual muscle fibers (microtrauma), either of which can cause the muscle to remain contracted over a long time; lack of oxygen from poor circulation; inflammation;

or mineral deposits in the muscle. Vitamin deficiencies, especially in vitamins B_1, B_6, B_{12}, and C, have been blamed by some for perpetuating TrPs, but not as yet for causing them.[6] Mineral deficiencies caused by poor absorption in the gut may actually cause trigger points.

If you want to feel around for trigger points yourself, start by locating the pain that is troubling you, then feel the muscles that lead toward that site. If one of these muscles contains an area that seems tight in comparison to others nearby, then you are probably close to your trigger point. This taut band of muscle fiber is caused by a shortening of the muscle's *sarcomeres,* horizontal segments of the vertical muscle fiber. Normal muscle functioning requires that all the sarcomeres remain the same length.

The significance of the shortened sarcomeres is that they are where the TrP will be found. Also, by understanding that taut muscles with foreshortened sarcomeres may be causing you pain, you will see the necessity of *gentle* stretching to restore the sarcomeres to their proper length. Forceful or sudden stretching is likely to result in the opposite of what you are trying to achieve; the muscle fibers can be torn, and the tighter they are the easier they are to tear. This is muscle microtrauma, one of the possible causes of your trigger point in the first place, and something you definitely want to avoid.

Trigger points do not have to be forever. It may be risky to try to stretch them out, but you can learn to apply pressure to a TrP and, possibly, release it. This is not easy, and it does hurt, so be warned. The pain may last a few minutes or a few days. Personally, I would never attempt something that might cause pain that lasts unless I did it on a weekend for which I had no important plans.

To differentiate between pain referred by TrPs and pain caused by pressure on a nerve, you should remember that trigger point pain is deep and aching, whereas compressed nerve pain is prickling, tingling, or numbing. Also, there are two kinds of TrPs, active and latent. An active trigger point is one that is currently causing episodes of referred pain. Pressing on it will duplicate the pain. A latent trigger point is not causing pain and will not send pain in response to pressure, although it may be tender. It may, however, cause a general *soreness* in the referred pain zone. If a needle is inserted into a latent trigger point, it will refer pain in the same way that an active trigger point does. It is possible, while poking around looking for trigger points, to activate a latent one. Overstretching muscles, repetitive motion or holding a position for an extended time, and chilling while the muscle is fatigued can also activate a latent TrP.

If you feel around for TrPs and try to release them, be sure that the spot you press is a myofascial *trigger* point and not a fibromyalgia *tender* point. Pressure on a tender point accomplishes nothing, and may leave you feeling needlessly sore. If you've found a trigger point (the muscle feels taut and ropy, it twitches, and refers pain to a site familiar to you for hurting), use the pads of your first two fingers to press on the point without moving, and hold the pressure for thirty seconds to two minutes, *until the pain lessens.* If, after two minutes, the pain is worse or no better, let up on the pressure and apply ice to the area to keep it from contracting even further. Later in this chapter is a discussion of various kinds of therapy for myofascial trigger points, some of which you can do yourself or with a partner, and some that require a trained professional.

Trigger Point Locations and Their Effects

Multivolume textbooks have been written on trigger point locations and the areas they affect (see Appendix A and "Background and Overview Articles"). It would be impossible to provide comprehensive information here. Instead, this section tells of some of the more common and accessible TrPs and the symptoms they can cause. It is important for you to understand that some kinds of pain may have more than one cause. For example, migraine headaches can be caused by a TrP, but TrPs are not always the cause of a particular migraine. Also, some symptoms can be caused by more than one trigger point; two trigger points can sometimes gang up on one location in the body. If this happens, both must be released before the pain will go away.

It can be difficult to determine whether a particular pain is caused by TrPs, fibromyalgia, or something entirely different. For example, pain in the lower right quadrant of the abdomen may be caused by gas, a trigger point, ovulation or a problem with the right ovary, by appendicitis, or by something else. If you have a persistent pain for which you can't find relief—and especially if that pain is accompanied by fever—do not try to treat yourself. I don't want to frighten you, but don't use your knowledge of trigger points to delay getting attention for something that is really wrong. Any time you are confronted by a new pain, it is important to stay calm so that you can think clearly about what has been going on, what is different in your life, your diet, your activities, and so on. It's all right to look for a trigger point and see if you can fix it yourself, but if your discomfort is severe, don't spend a lot of time at it before you get help.

Here are a few of the common types of pain and their associated trigger points.

• Migraine or severe tension headache: If the pain is on the top of your head, find the muscle band that runs from the top of your shoulder up the back of your neck to the base of your skull. If there is a trigger point, it should be the width of about three fingers from the bottom of your skull.

• If the headache is worse at your temple, find the muscle band that runs diagonally from behind your collarbone to behind your ear. The trigger point should be about an inch below the corner of your jaw.

• Earache: may be caused by the same TrP that causes a headache in the temple.

• Shoulder pain: Place your fingers at the margin between the front of your shoulder and your upper chest. You may find a TrP there.

• Breast pain: Find the muscle at the outer top of the breast that moves when you raise your arm out and to the side. Look for a trigger point at its lower edge.

• Heel pain: Run your finger up the Achilles tendon and onto the calf muscle. The TrP may be about an inch above where the muscle begins.

• Carpal tunnel–type pain: Press gently under your arm toward the back, just in front of the lower point of the shoulder blade.

• Urinary urgency and irritable bowel syndrome may be caused by TrPs deep in the abdomen, just above the pubic bone.

• Toe pain that feels like gout may be caused by a TrP an inch or two below the knee, just about where a kneehigh stocking ends.

Therapy for Myofascial Pain

Trigger points may be treated by injection, massage, or by a method known as spray and stretch. Trigger point injections may contain a local anesthetic such as lidocaine. Some doctors will include cortisone in the injection if they suspect there is inflammation. One clinical study found that inserting a dry needle into the trigger point, injecting nothing, was just as effective in relieving the TrP. Regardless of the technique, the affected area may be more painful and the surrounding muscles more sore for up to forty-eight hours after treatment by injection.

Some physicians will suggest a myofascial massage either before or just after a trigger point injection. If the massage is done right after an injection of a local anesthetic, it is easier to stretch the muscles and help them regain some of their former elasticity. You should ask to be shown some gentle exercises that you can do at home to improve the functioning of the muscle and prevent the return of the trigger point.

Even without injections, myofascial massage is worth considering. Some people who have undergone this form of therapy report that they go through a couple of days of what they describe as flulike symptoms after a massage, but that afterward the trigger points that have been worked on are gone, as is the associated referred pain. It is critical to find a massage therapist who really understands myofascial pain and knows the proper technique for releasing trigger points.

Be prepared: Myofascial release hurts. Pressure that is firm enough to release the TrP is often hard enough to cause real pain. You need to work with a massage therapist who will respect your right to have the final word on how much pain you can stand. If you think of pain as being on a ten-point scale, where one is mere discomfort and ten is the worst pain you've ever had, you may need to go as far as an eight to get significant trigger point release. You will probably find that you reach an eight sooner as the session continues, your resistance to pain having decreased.

There is a school of thought concerning myofascial massage that believes that pain during massage comes from the resistance of the person being massaged. I think this approach is all wrong for people with fibromyalgia. The other approach is closer to the Shiatsu technique, following energy meridians, with firm, slow strokes, hovering around trigger points when they are discovered, to the limit of your tolerance. If the pressure is too hard, the practitioner will ease up somewhat, but will continue working near the TrP until it releases. If you say, "That's enough there," and the therapist doesn't listen, find another therapist.

Telling about her experience with myofascial massage, one woman said, "I'm convinced that the only reason I'm not twisted into a pretzel shape is because I get massaged regularly. The first few sessions can be intense, but as the points get cleared out, you can feel your muscles unkinking with each visit. It's definitely worth it."

Keep in mind that myofascial release massage breaks up places in the muscle where metabolic wastes have accumulated.

This is the reason that many people say they experience a day or two of flulike aches after a massage session. One way to minimize the discomfort is to drink plenty of pure water to help wash the toxins away. Another comforting after-massage technique is to take an Epsom salts bath. Pour half a milk-carton box of Epsom salts into a tub of the hottest water you can stand, and soak in the tub for twenty minutes, then rinse off with lukewarm water. This promotes sweating; since your skin is the largest organ of elimination, you will get rid of the released toxins more quickly. Be sure to take a bottle of drinking water into the bathroom with you; believe it or not, you can become dehydrated sitting in a tub of Epsom salts water.

Dry brushing also helps get rid of the toxins by stimulating the lymph system, which carries away waste products. Using a long-handled dry bath brush, brush upward on your legs and arms, toward your heart. Start gently, and as you get more accustomed to the feeling, brush more briskly.

Craniosacral release is another kind of massage, often used in conjunction with myofascial release. Its purpose is to release tension stored in the connective tissues. A very gentle form of massage therapy, it is based on the theory that restrictive tensions resulting from infection, inflammation, and various other conditions block the energy in the connective tissue that causes motion. Physical therapists are often trained in both forms of massage.

For people who are bedridden or nearly so, lymphatic massage may be a good place to start. The lymphatic system is a primitive sort of circulatory system. It consists of lymph glands, or nodes, located throughout the body; the most noticeable are in the armpits and groin. There are also small blood vessel–like tubes called the lymphatics that link the lymph nodes and the spleen, a large lymph gland located in the upper left quadrant of the abdomen behind the ribs.

The lymph nodes produce lymphocytes, a form of white blood cell whose purpose is to recognize foreign substances such as infectious agents and mount a battle against them. They are our body's first line of defense against the spread of infection.

Often, if you are fighting an infection, the lymph nodes become swollen because they are trapping the infectious agents.

When it is not busy fighting infection, the lymphatic system carries the waste products of muscle metabolism through the lymph nodes and into the bloodstream. The lymph nodes act as one-way valves; the lymph fluid pushes them open and passes through on the way to being transferred into the bloodstream. The kidneys filter the wastes from the blood and excrete them from the body in the urine.

Unlike the blood circulatory system, the lymph system has no heart to act as a pump and keep lymph fluids moving, so it must rely on body motion to help it do its work. If you are inactive, the lymph system is apt to slow down or even stop its circulating action. If this happens, the lymph vessels fill up with unreleased wastes, which may swell and harden; they may even become painful.

In lymphatic massage, the practitioner pushes gently along the lymph vessels toward the nodes, making the fluid move and sending the wastes on their way to the kidneys and then out the body. The massage itself should not be painful. Depending on how long the lymph system has been blocked, there may be a great deal of waste dumped into the kidneys, and you may find yourself urinating much more frequently for a few hours after a massage session.

Once the lymphatic fluid has begun to flow freely, it should continue to do so unless you become immobilized again. It doesn't take a great deal of motion to keep the lymph flowing. Even people with sedentary occupations stimulate sufficient lymph activity, but people who are bedridden may not.

As with other forms of massage, it is important to drink plenty of water. If you have been taking medications whose residues have been trapped in your lymph system, you may feel groggy for a few hours after the session as these drug residues move on to excretion by the kidneys. Excessive urination and grogginess, as well as a feeling of relaxation, are all signs that the lymphatic massage is working.

Writing about lymphatic massage, one woman says this:

> I had fibromyalgia for three years before I found lymphatic massage. Nothing else that I tried had helped, except for pain medications. My lymph vessels were so hard and swollen that I could see them through the skin, when shown where to look. My first massage was very gentle and lasted about thirty minutes. Afterward, I had the dopey feeling and needed to urinate frequently, but the next day, it hit. It felt like a bad case of food poisoning. Everything inside me came out, one way or another, and I felt totally drugged for about two more days. Then the fog lifted and I felt better. Within three treatments, my massage therapist was combining deep muscle massage, pushing with her body weight, with lymphatic work. My muscle and joint pain decreased by about 50 percent, and pain medications were reduced by about the same. The aftereffects now are simply increased urination and slight grogginess.

Spray and stretch therapy is another treatment often used to relieve myofascial pain. The therapist uses a coolant spray, administering it to the skin and directing the spray from the trigger point to the area of referred pain, and then stretching the affected muscle. People who have had this treatment report relief from pain and increased range of motion lasting from a few hours to several days or even longer. A period of conscious muscle relaxation should precede the spraying. The coolant spray, which can cause frostbite in the hands of a careless therapist, shuts off the pain centers of the brain for a brief period, during which the therapist can take advantage of the opportunity to stretch the muscle to its normal length. In the process, the trigger point may be released.

CASE HISTORY: SALLY, 54, RETIRED RESEARCHER

Sally has a doctoral degree in sociology and used to work as a researcher in the health care field. She left her job, thinking she was just "burned out." She had seen one doctor after another for years, with a variety of diagnoses and no relief. She now stays home and keeps house.

In her teens, Sally says she had "growing pains," now generally recognized as an indicator of a predisposition toward fibromyalgia. Her other symptoms—fatigue, headaches, ear pain, poor memory, muscle cramps in her legs and feet, and hypoglycemia—began when she was thirty-four and in a highly stressful job. Sally was fifty-one when a rheumatologist interested in fibromyalgia research diagnosed her FM.

Sally says her ability to concentrate and to draw upon her memory comes and goes. She has the pain of carpal tunnel syndrome (CTS) that cannot be verified with diagnostic tests. She is extremely susceptible to stress, and sensitive to light and noise. Sally has both an irritable bowel, alternating between diarrhea and constipation, and an irritable bladder; she often feels the urgent need to urinate, even though her bladder is not nearly full. She had endometriosis, but says that "menopause has cleared that up." Her sleep is light and hardly refreshing, even though she is taking a small dose of tricyclic antidepressant to combat alpha-wave intrusion in her deep-level sleep. Like many people who have fibromyalgia, Sally has "permanent goosebumps" on her upper arms and legs. Her fingernails show pronounced vertical ridges, another sign common among fibromyalgics. Physical therapy has helped greatly with her low back pain and sciatica.

Sally says her husband has generally denied that anything was wrong with her, but not in an unpleasant way. Recently, she has spent a significant amount of time learning about fibromyalgia. She says, "Now that I am clearer about what is going on with this condition, I can state more clearly what my needs are in a matter-of-fact manner, and we both just accept it.

"I am not terribly disabled," she adds. "I can cook, get groceries, clean, and do some socializing, so it's not as big a deal as it is with some people." Nonetheless, Sally has streamlined her life. "I have cut back on the amount of housecleaning I do," she says, "and I have simplified meal preparation with easy recipes." She holds back from social and civic activities because "I get so tired of telling people that I am too tired to do things, so I don't get involved in the first place," she says. "I promise very little and often regret even those few promises I do make. I read a lot, garden, talk by phone, and write letters. And I have a few friends that I see once a week, if I feel up to it."

When people ask why she won't join them in some activity, Sally tells all. "I don't like the feeling of pity that I get from some of them, but I just can't lie about it. I feel kind of belligerent about it, I guess," she says.

Sally has a word of advice for people with fibromyalgia who are having trouble in their sex lives. "Develop a broad view of what sex is," she suggests. "Hugging, touching, and holding are all important parts of sex, too."

CHAPTER SIX

Theories About the Causes of Fibromyalgia

Do you remember the legend about the blind men and the elephant? Each one had his hands on a different part of the animal, and they were arguing about what it was. One, holding the tail, said the elephant was a rope. Another, with his hands on the elephant's leg, said it was a tree. A third, touching the elephant's side, said it was a wall. Each had a part of the truth, but none could see the whole animal.

Fibromyalgia is a lot like that elephant. Each of us who has FM experiences it slightly differently, depending on which symptoms we find most distressing. For me, fibromyalgia is a sleep disturbance; if I can sleep well, pain recedes into the background. Others, who have more pain than I do, see their lack of restorative sleep as a consequence of the pain. There are probably as many ways of describing fibromyalgia as there are symptoms that make up the syndrome. Each of us has a part of the truth, but none of us sees the whole disorder.

Indeed, this is also true of the doctors who research FM and those who treat it, only their views are defined not by the symptoms they experience but by their area of specialty. Each researcher studies some aspect of the disorder and finds something that most people with fibromyalgia have in common. We know, for example, that many fibromyalgics have too much substance P, a chemical that receives pain messages, and too little serotonin, a chemical that dulls the perception of pain. We know several things of this sort, but none applies to all people with fibromyalgia, and none explains *why* these things are true, when they are true.

This is not a criticism of those who are doing FM research. If they didn't have an area of specialization in which to do the research, they wouldn't be researchers at all. We need them to continue their work, and to publish what they find out so that we can all understand more about this vexing condition. But we also need generalists—people who know about many things, but not to the depth of a specialist's knowledge. This is the role of a primary care physician and of people like you and me, who can gather in the conclusions of FM research projects and perhaps see them as a whole, not as parts of the FM elephant.

Sleep Theories

In 1975, Dr. Harvey Moldofsky induced the fibromyalgia syndrome, complete with tender points, in healthy volunteers by preventing them from getting slow-wave sleep.[7] All of the volunteers recovered from their symptoms when they were allowed to sleep normally. People with FM don't seem to recover from it fully, although most get better once they find the program that works for them. What makes some people who are deprived of sleep get FM while others do not? There is evidence that FM tends to run in families, but that doesn't explain what happens in an individual body that makes it develop FM. Nor is there any compelling information on what makes alpha waves intrude into delta sleep—in other words, what causes the sleep disturbance when there's no one around to wake us up. Also, there are people who have alpha-delta sleep dysfunction and don't have fibromyalgia. Apparently, sleep dysfunction is not sufficient to cause FM.

Chemical Disturbances

It's well known that you're more likely to get sick if you're run-down, overstressed, and lacking sleep. Something changes in your body at such times. Those changes are brought about by the action or inaction of your immune system. Like everything else in your body, your immune system is made up of chemicals that have different purposes in maintaining the goal of all beings: homeostasis, which means keeping things on an even keel.

For example, your body likes to operate within a certain temperature range. If your temperature goes too low, certain chemicals swing into action to bring it back up. Chemicals bear the messages to all parts of your body, telling your muscles to shiver and your heart to work harder to move your blood around faster.

For the most part, the chemicals suspected of causing FM distress are called neurotransmitters, or neurohormones. These are the brain's chemical messengers. Their action is so interrelated that it is impossible to point to one and say, "Here, this is the neurotransmitter that is causing all your problems." But looking at what is known about their actions may provide some clues.

For this discussion, we can confine our attention to a few neurotransmitters, serotonin in particular. Increasing its availability leads to a reduction in symptoms in many people who have fibromyalgia, but it is not clear whether the result comes from better sleep or an increased ability to tolerate pain.

Epinephrine and norepinephrine are also important. Many people with FM experience a flare-up of symptoms or at least exaggerated fatigue following any stimulus that results in the sudden discharge of these neurotransmitters.[8] I have discovered that I can minimize this effect through vigorous exercise (or what is vigorous for me) for a while after something happens that makes my system pump adrenaline (another name for epinephrine). I thought I was "burning off" excess adrenaline, until I read a study that found lower concentrations of epinephrine in people with fibromyalgia after they exercised to the point of exhaustion, as compared with study subjects who had no FM diagnosis. Heart rates were also lower in the fibromyalgics. The researchers suggest that the higher concentration of the excitatory neurotransmitters, coupled with the lower heart rate, may indicate an overreactive nervous system in people who have fibromyalgia. Another FM researcher found that the cells of 40 percent of the people he tested had more than the normal number of receptors for these neurotransmitters, which could explain an exaggerated response to stress. Raynaud's phenomenon and the tendency that many of us have for the blood vessels in our hands and feet to go into spasms when we are cold are two more pieces of this puzzle.

Digestive Disturbance

Let's assume, for the moment, that our problems come from a disturbance in the amounts of various neurotransmitters in our nervous system. The obvious question then is why does this happen and, if we can figure that out, what can be done about it? Of course, some of us are already taking medicines to correct the deficiency in serotonin: tricyclic agents such as amitriptyline (Elavil), and 5-hydroxytryptophan (5-htp), a breakdown product of the amino acid tryptophan and a precursor of serotonin. But replacing a missing substance is not the same as helping the body to produce sufficient quantities by itself. To do this, we need to know the reason the deficiency exists.

One theory has to do with our ability to digest the nutrients in the food we eat. Most of the neurotransmission chemicals in the brain are composed of amino acids, the building blocks of the proteins that make up our bodies. We get amino acids from the foods we eat. Different foods contain different combinations and quantities of amino acids. No single food has all of the amino acids we require in the proportions that we require them, which is why we are advised to eat a wide variety of foods. Turkey has the most complete collection of amino acids of any food consumed by human beings. The combination of beans and rice provides another nearly complete amino acid chain. Excess amino acids, or amino acids that cannot find the others needed to form a complete chain, are excreted in the urine or passed as intestinal gas.

Neurotransmitters are made from amino acids; tryptophan becomes serotonin, epinephrine and norepinephrine are derived from the amino acid tyrosine. In 1988, FM researcher I. Jon Russell, M.D., measured amino acid levels in the blood serum of twenty people who have fibromyalgia and compared the results to an equal number of healthy subjects. Tryptophan and six other essential amino acids (alanine, histidine, lysine, proline, serine, and threonine) were found to be low. Perhaps, he reasoned, the digestive system in fibromyalgics fails to absorb the amino acids from our foods efficiently.

Judging from conversations with many people who have fibromyalgia, there is evidence to suggest that these people do not absorb other nutrients well, but no scientific studies in this area have been reported. For example, a significant number of people who seem to have carpal tunnel syndrome or have joint pain suggesting arthritis find that their symptoms disappear when they increase their intake of vitamin B_6 (pyridoxine), which contributes to nerve health. Vitamin B_6 also takes part in the process of turning the amino acid tryptophan into serotonin. If people with FM don't absorb vitamins and amino acids well, that might explain some of the neurotransmitter problems that we have. It could also explain why different people who have fibromyalgia seem to have problems with different neurotransmitters.

Immune System Abnormalities

Usually, when people think of a problem with the immune system, they think of either an underactive immune system in which the person is more susceptible to illness or an autoimmune disease, in which the body is attacked by its own immune system. There is no evidence that either of these situations pertains to fibromyalgia. But there is evidence that the immune system is involved in some way.

The immune system is made up of a variety of chemical substances that normally work to surround and destroy invading matter such as infectious agents and poisons. Coordinating the activities of the immune system chemicals is a group of hormonelike substances known as cytokines. Interleukin and interferon are two classes of cytokines. Serotonin plays a role in this process of cytokine production, too. It also appears that sleep, or the lack of sleep, has an effect on the functioning of the immune system, possibly because the growth hormone secreted during deep sleep affects the production of cytokines. One theory holds that one of the by-products of growth hormone serves to slow the production of cytokines. If this is so, then it could explain why FM, particularly in the early stages, feels like a bad case of the flu.

Many symptoms of the flu and other contagious illnesses that make us want to stay in bed are caused by the presence of an overload of cytokines, produced as part of the body's attempt to overwhelm the invading infectious agents and help us get well. It appears that the cytokine-damping function is flawed in people who have fibromyalgia, because their sleep disturbance fails to stop the process of producing cytokines even after the initial illness is gone.

Another possibility is that cortisol, a hormone that controls the level of activity of the immune system, is to blame. Too much cortisol is thought to lead to suppression of immune system activity, while too little cortisol allows the immune system to become overactive. Some studies have found that people with fibromyalgia have too little cortisol, which, according to this line of reasoning, leads to an overactive immune system. Overactive, however, does not mean stronger nor does it suggest that FM is an autoimmune disease, in which the immune system attacks instead of protects the body.

The Limbic System and the HPA Axis

Increasingly researchers are blaming the central nervous system for the symptoms that make up the fibromyalgia syndrome. The central nervous system is composed of the brain and spinal cord, the hub of the network that coordinates and controls our bodies. The parts of the brain of greatest interest to FM researchers are the limbic system and the hypothalamus. Anatomy teachers consider the hypothalamus to be separate from the limbic system, but in terms of the brain's functioning it is a central part of the limbic system.

Some researchers think the underlying cause of fibromyalgia can be found in the limbic system; others are exploring the interaction of the hypothalamus and the pituitary and adrenal glands—the hypothalamic-pituitary-adrenal or HPA axis. The pituitary gland sits at the back of the hypothalamus, and the adrenal glands are located on top of the kidneys. The hypothalamus contains centers for regulating body temperature, blood pressure, pulse rate, perspiration, the release or retention of fluids, and other functions controlled by the autonomic (involuntary) nervous system. It also regulates the production and release of hormones. The limbic system is associated with memory and emotion. You can see how a disturbance in this area could cause virtually all of the problems that we experience with FM.

There are two classes of theory concerning the limbic system and HPA axis. One suggests the presence of a virus, the other proposes that dysfunction is the physical result of extended mental stress. This is not the same as saying that fibromyalgia is all in your head. Scientists have shown that sending the same signal repeatedly over the same nerve path will eventually cause alterations in the nerve path itself. The question we need answers to is this: If something has altered the nerve paths such that we experience so many different and confusing symptoms, what can be done about it? Experiments are under way; perhaps we'll have an answer before long.

Phosphate Metabolism

For several years, one doctor, Paul St. Amand, has been treating people with FM by prescribing a common substance normally used in cough medicines. The theory has been tested in a one-year clinical trial. Unfortunately, the results will not be published until after this book goes to press. At the time this was written no one, not even the physician who supervised the experiment, knew what the results would show. Some people who have tried it outside the experiment say the treatment has helped them greatly. Others say it has made no difference in their condition. One of the reasons the results may vary from person to person or group to group is we still do not know whether all people who have fibromyalgia's symptoms have the same disorder, caused by the same malfunction.

St. Amand is an endocrinologist, a gland specialist. Because endocrinologists focus on metabolic disorders—problems in the way the body processes nourishment—they tend to look at the body as a huge chemical factory. We take in food and use the chemicals that our bodies manufacture from it to make body tissues and energy, and more chemicals to manufacture more tissues and energy. What we eat, and the way we process it, is critical to our well-being.

St. Amand's theory is that fibromyalgics have an inherited abnormality in the ability to excrete phosphates, which are present in almost everything we eat. In normally healthy people, excess phosphates are carried off by the kidneys. In people who have fibromyalgia, he thinks, phosphates accumulate within our cells, specifically in the portion of the cells called mitochondria, the body's energy factories.

St. Amand treats his fibromyalgia patients with guaifenesin (gwai-FEN-uh-sin), a common ingredient in cough medicines. Guaifenesin loosens mucus and is commonly used by patients with chronic sinusitis. It also seems to increase the excretion of phosphates. Although guaifenesin has been used for generations, no harmful side effects have yet been discovered. However, no one has taken guaifenesin over a long period in doses as large as those used in this treatment, so long-term side effects are possible.

The theory is that phosphates get stored in the cells and build up in different places in the body, causing a variety of symptoms. St. Amand first examines a patient, mapping on an outline drawing of the human body all the places where the patient feels pain. He prescribes doses ranging from a beginning

300 mg of guaifenesin to as much as 2,400 mg, depending on how the person responds to the smaller dose.

The treatment can be unpleasant at times. Most people experience a few days of flulike symptoms within a few days of taking the first dose of guaifenesin. This, according to St. Amand, is a sign that the phosphate deposits are beginning to dissolve. There follows a succession of good days, followed by bad days, and the cycle repeats itself. Gradually, the good days outnumber the bad days.

Typically, according to St. Amand, deposits dissolve in reverse order to the way they accumulated. As the deposits in a particular area dissolve, the symptoms associated with that area repeat themselves, then go away for good. St. Amand estimates that it takes about six weeks of guaifenesin treatment to reverse a year's worth of phosphate deposits. If this is so, then it follows that the sooner treatment begins, the sooner the deposits will be gone.

Eventually, if the treatment works, all deposits will be gone, symptoms will be gone, and all that will be required is a maintenance dose of guaifenesin to prevent the deposits from building up again.

An interesting sidelight: Paul St. Amand has FM himself and has been taking guaifenesin for several years. He says it has worked for him (you will find contact information in Appendix A). Dr. St. Amand is willing to discuss this therapy with other doctors.

CASE HISTORY: FRANCES, 45, COMPUTER PROGRAMMER/ANALYST

Frances links the onset of fibromyalgia with three simultaneous and stressful events in her life. Her employer announced that her job was being discontinued and assigned her to training to become a computer programmer. Her teenage son ran afoul of the law. And Frances fell down a flight of stairs. She began experiencing pain in her neck and shoulders, which soon traveled down her arms and left her hands numb. Then her legs started to hurt, she developed a constant headache, and irritable bowel syndrome began to plague her. Her physician treated each of these symptoms as an individual problem, never considering them as a syndrome. Pain pills made her sleepy, but did not relieve the pain. Frances got the flu that was making its way through her programming class, and couldn't seem to recover.

Her doctor sent her to a neurologist, who hospitalized her and ordered a battery of tests, all of which revealed nothing. "Then they sent in the psychiatrist," Frances says. "I knew I didn't need psychiatric treatment, so I started looking for another doctor." Five doctors and eighteen months later, she saw "a female internist who spent fifteen minutes talking to me and then asked if I had ever heard of fibromyalgia." The doctor prescribed Elavil (amitriptyline) and an NSAID. "After six months of experimenting with dosages, I reached a level where I could cope with the pain and symptoms," she says.

Frances says her reaction to being diagnosed with FM was anger. "I was very angry that I had something that could not be cured, and angry that it took three years of escalating pain to get help. There was also a lot of grief, and the need to decide how I was going to live with it," she recalls, adding, "I also had to try to restore some relationships that had been damaged by my health problem."

Today, Frances says that the worst part of her FM is cognitive difficulty, which fluctuates along with her pain symptoms. "This is the most frustrating of all, because it affects my job the most, adding fear of losing my way of earning a living, and decreasing my self-confidence."

Frances doesn't talk about her condition much, even with family members. "I try not to complain, and they remember I have FM only when I have attacks where it becomes noticeable and I can't keep going on normally," she says. Her husband, she says, helps her with heavy work around the house, and with anything that requires working with raised arms, such as changing overhead light bulbs. "He's great about helping, and does what I ask him to do. He knows why I ask without my telling him," she adds.

She says she was much more socially active before FM began than she is now, but she still goes out with friends when she feels up to it, and attends adult education classes that interest her. Mostly, however, she turns down invitations and requests for volunteer work. "If I do commit to something, I do so knowing I am not central to the task, either mentally or physically," she says.

Frances has not told her employer or co-workers about her fibromyalgia, because she is afraid of discrimination against her. The company allows employees to take sick leave for no more than five different illnesses within any twelve-month period. "I come to work when I'm in a lot of pain. Only the diarrhea stops me," she says. She worries about days on which she is less than normally productive, and tries to make up for the bad days when she has good ones.

Even so, Frances says that having FM is not all bad. "In some ways it has made my husband and me closer to each other. He was very frightened before I was diagnosed," she says. "He let me know how he felt all along the way, so I had to let him know how I felt. Now we don't have to talk about it much; he can read me, and I can read him."

The worst part, she says, is that she has hardly any sex drive left. Her solution is simple: "Talk about it. I think the most helpful thing for my husband was when I finally explained it well enough that he understood it has nothing to do with him," she says. "The most handsome movie star in the world could be standing in front of me and I wouldn't react, so it's certainly no reflection on my feelings about my husband. Once he understood that, the problem was gone."

CHAPTER SEVEN

Fibromyalgia in Children

UNTIL recently, fibromyalgia was considered an adult disorder. Then, in a study published in the *Journal of Rheumatology* in 1993, a team of doctors in Israel reported that 6.2 percent of 338 healthy schoolchildren between the ages of nine and fifteen met the criteria for the fibromyalgia syndrome.[9] At nearly the same time, a rheumatologist in the United States asserted that 45 percent of the children referred to him had FM.[10] Of these fifteen children, nine had been diagnosed incorrectly with juvenile chronic arthritis, three had been told they had growing pains, and two had been given a psychiatric diagnosis.

Since then, doctors have been paying more attention to children's complaints of pain and are diagnosing FM with increasing frequency. As awareness grows, it seems quite likely that FM will be found in children in a proportion comparable to that of the population as a whole.

Children's complaints of pain must be taken seriously, lest they grow up with untreated FM. Growing pains are a particularly pernicious myth. It should not hurt to grow, and the child whose pain is brushed off that way is an unfortunate person.

FM is often a family affair. In a 1989 study of seventeen people with fibromyalgia and fifty of their parents and siblings, 52 percent of the relatives had FM. Of those not affected, 22 percent had the ropy muscles characteristic of FM but no tender points.[11] That is *not* to say that your children are sure to have FM if you do—and some children may mimic the pain behavior of their elders—but be extra vigilant in taking seriously children's complaints of pain. Fibromyalgia can make a child's life miserable at school and on the playground. The child with FM needs a great deal of special help and understanding.

Many adults think of childhood as a carefree time, full of fun and excitement. Some find it hard to comprehend the depth to which children can feel pain, both emotional and physical. Small children want nothing so much as to please the adults around them, and to gain their respect and affection. If parents place a high value on stoicism, then their child will believe that the way to gain approval is to grin and bear it, and is likely to miss badly needed medical attention.

Detecting FM in Children

FM in children often starts with a flulike illness from which the child seems never to fully recover. Sometimes, particularly in children before puberty, FM simply comes on gradually, without any obvious precipitating event.

Very young children may not remember a time without pain, and thus may not complain at all. As in adults, childhood fibromyalgia may mimic some other ailment. One team of doctors wrote of seeing a large number of children with FM who had been incorrectly diagnosed as having Lyme disease.[12]

You should suspect fibromyalgia in a child who sleeps restlessly, kicks or twitches during sleep, and has a difficult time getting out of bed in the morning. One mother said her three-year-old son, after having had insomnia for a few months, was complaining of aches in his legs. It is not unusual for a three-year-old to wake up at night needing to go to the bathroom but not realizing it, or because of a bad dream, but insomnia coupled with pains or aches is a trouble signal and should not be ignored, particularly if one of the child's parents has FM.

Sometimes an alert teacher is the first to notice a problem. One teacher described a ten-year-old boy who suffered from unexplained stomach pain; his diagnostic tests showed him to be normal, but the pain, he said, "feels like someone is inside cutting me." He told his teacher he went to bed at 10:00, but often didn't get to sleep until 2:00 A.M. and still felt tired when he woke up in the morning. There are other reasons why a child might feel this way, but FM should certainly be considered.

Children with fibromyalgia often have trouble in school. A considerable amount of schoolwork requires memorization. The cognitive difficulties that often accompany FM may make this difficult, if not impossible. One high school student said: "I am having memory problems. I'm too young to be as forgetful as I am. I've always been an excellent student, until the past two years. I've had to drop certain classes because I don't seem to have the capacity to remember simple things. School has grown much harder, and I have to spend hours doing what used to take me a few minutes. I'm looking forward to college, but I'm getting more and more worried."

Recalling her high school years, a college freshman told me: "My most difficult problems in high school were memorizing words for vocabulary tests and memorizing my lines for plays. I never did figure out a system for the vocabulary tests, but I did work with my director a lot on memorization to help me get through my last two plays in high school. Since going to college, I've ignored the problem more than I've faced it. I tried to take Russian last fall, but it was eating up almost six hours a day of studying and I still barely understood anything. I dropped the class after about four weeks. I know that my brain just won't engage that way right now. I still have the fogginess, but I try to avoid involvement in activities in which fogginess would be a problem."

FM for me as a child consisted of intermittent severe diarrhea, difficulty controlling my bladder, shooting pains in my legs, deep aches in my calf muscles that felt as though my marrow was burning, frequent severe headaches, lack of stamina, and insomnia. Some of my earliest school memories are of teachers joining in with my classmates to taunt me because I was awkward and had poor coordination. Needless to say, I was never the first chosen for any team game. I can't remember being aware of tender points except on my knees. That made kneeling intolerably painful, which in turn made it impossible for me to participate in many of the games that were popular at that time.

Children who squirm and fidget in class may be trying to keep themselves from falling asleep. They may also find it painful to sit in one place for long periods of time. Some symptoms of FM may manifest themselves in the classroom as attention deficit disorder (ADD). Not all children with ADD are hyperactive, as was once thought. There is a form known as quiet-ADD. Some pediatricians say this may be an early symptom of fibromyalgia in some children.[13] A sharp pediatrician can tell the difference between ADD and FM by performing a tender point examination.

Many children with FM, like their elders, find it difficult to hold a pencil or pen. Often, their handwriting is terrible. Particularly in the elementary grades, teachers place great emphasis on handwriting and may penalize a child with FM for handing in untidily written papers.

Another characteristic of children with fibromyalgia is that many of them have hypermobile joints, that is, they are "double-jointed."[14] One woman, looking back on her childhood, recalled, "Double-jointedness was a problem when I was learning to write. My handwriting is still not good. It also made me somewhat of a novelty, providing many laughs for my peers. I could actually sit cross-legged on the floor, then lift my ankles up behind my neck." Being double-jointed is not a sure sign of FM, but it should make a parent suspicious.

All parents, particularly those with FM, should see to it that their children are examined for fibromyalgia as soon as they are old enough to say if they feel pain during a tender point examination. Early intervention is important; proper treatment may save the child from a lifetime of suffering. Some doctors put children with FM on a very small dose of a tricyclic agent or muscle relaxant. Others prescribe Benadryl at bedtime for sleep. A child who learns good nutritional habits early in life, who grows accustomed to going to bed at the same time every night, and who is encouraged to take part in a suitable exercise program will be well equipped to avoid FM flare-ups throughout life.

If your child is diagnosed with FM, you will need to do some explaining. What you say and how you say it will have a profound effect on the child's reaction. Children are particularly vulnerable to thinking that anything that goes wrong is their fault. You must stress that FM is nobody's fault and that nothing anyone could have done would have prevented it. How much you explain about fibromyalgia will depend, of course, on the child's age and intellectual development. Above all, the child must understand that FM can be controlled.

Children hate anything that sets them apart from their agemates. Said one young woman, "The hardest part about being a sick kid is the feeling that you're different from everybody else and that difference is a bad thing." It may be helpful if you explain to your child that no one's body is perfect, and that everyone is different in one way or another. I learned this in a college anatomy class, and it changed completely my view of my own physical shortcomings.

Raising a child who has fibromyalgia is a real challenge. You will need to remember that some days are worse than others, and allow the child to set the pace. Household chores should be adjusted to fit the situation, and flexibility should be the overriding principle.

Teachers and school administrators should be informed about your child's FM. They must understand that the child can feel well one day and terrible the next, and that people with fibromyalgia almost always look better than they feel. One mother sent the following letter to her daughter's middle school teachers. You can use this letter as a sample, and adapt it to your child's particular symptoms.

Dear Teacher,

This is to inform you that my daughter, [name], is under her physician's care for a medical condition known as fibromyalgia. The symptoms of this condition include widespread pain, headaches, urinary and bowel problems, and a sleep disturbance. There is no known cure, but remission is possible, and that is the goal of treatment. Fibromyalgia is not life-threatening.

I ask for your understanding and hope that this short explanation will help if she complains and needs to go to the nurse, or use the restroom or the elevator. She may, from time to time, need to use crutches or a wheelchair. The pain will move around; she may experience knee pain one day and back pain the next, as well as a variety of other symptoms. Just where the pain will strike at any given time is unpredictable.

I would welcome the opportunity to provide you with more detailed information if you wish. [The school nurse's name] is fully aware of the situation and can fill you in as well. I know that [child's name] will do her very best in school even under these conditions. While [child's name] would be happy to discuss this with you, I'm sure she would prefer a private setting should you wish to inquire about her health.

Please do not hesitate to call if you have any questions. Our phone number is [XXX-XXXX].

Sincerely,
[Your name]

Any condition that interferes with a child's learning ability entitles the child to a special needs assessment and education plan, according to U.S. Public Law 94-142, which provides for the education of children with special needs. If your child is having trouble with schoolwork, you may have to be persistent in getting the school to agree to this assessment, but it is your right and you will eventually prevail if you keep at it. Among the accommodations that have been granted to children with FM are two sets of school books so that the child need not carry books to and from school; a tape recorder to eliminate the need to take notes; and a flexible class schedule that allows the child to take her most difficult classes at the time of day when she is feeling her best. If your child's classmates are making his or her life miserable with teasing, a word with the teacher is in order. Children generally take their behavior cues from their teachers. If the teacher makes an offhand remark about the FM child's clumsiness, or chides the child for being lazy when fatigue strikes, the teacher's attitude will surely lead to teasing by the other children. It is up to you to cultivate the kind of relationship in which your child can confide in you about such problems. An appointment with the school's guidance counselor can often set things right.

Proper treatment can make a world of difference. One mother, after struggling to find medical care that would help her son, and pushing the public school until a suitable education plan was established, told me: "He has gone from being unable to attend school for the majority of the last semester to getting up daily and being able to play basketball with his friends every other day. He now has a positive attitude and doctors who listen to him and believe him. They have helped him in learning how to cope with the daily pain."

There is evidence that fibromyalgia in children may not be a lifetime sentence. One study found that thirty months after diagnosis, eleven of fifteen children with FM (73 percent) were no longer fibromyalgic. "We suggest that the outcome of FM in children is more favorable than in adults," the doctors who conducted the study wrote. Guaifenesin has been found to bring some children to a pain-free state, according to their parents. Early intervention seems to be the key in children with fibromyalgia.

CASE HISTORY: ALICIA, 19, COLLEGE STUDENT

From the perspective of a junior in college, Alicia looks back at her early years as a time of horror. Shopping with her parents at the age of five, her legs and arms would hurt so badly she would beg to be carried. She also showed signs of hypoglycemia, but it went unrecognized. "If I didn't eat right, I would get mean. I'd start to shake, and snap and yell at people," she says. "They tested me for diabetes. I bruised easily, so they tested me for leukemia." She had no idea that her pain was unusual, so she didn't often mention it.

A couple of years later, she failed the Presidential fitness exam because she couldn't chin herself. The gym teacher had lifted her so that she could hang from the chinning bar, but Alicia could neither pull herself up nor drop to the floor. "I was afraid to drop because I had very weak ankles and I knew it would hurt," she says. "I just hung there and screamed for the teacher to get me down." The teacher called Alicia's mother. "She told her that I was a rude and obstinate child," Alicia recalls.

Her classmates teased her. She was the first to get hit in dodge ball, because she had neither the coordination nor the speed to get out of the way. And getting hit by the ball hurt. "It was so easy to tease me. All they had to do was to hit me with the ball and I would start crying. My entire body would hurt," she says. "I had no friends in elementary school. They all thought I was a hypochondriac."

Alicia slept poorly at night, but she fell asleep at awkward times. "Many times I fell asleep during recess, or during class. The doctor blamed it on ear infections or strep infections and things like that," she says. She needed to urinate frequently, which meant getting an adult to unlock the restroom door for her. "I had to go to the bathroom so many times a day that I was embarrassed, so I started holding my urine from the time I left home until I got home again. Then I started wetting my pants on the bus ride home. I didn't drink much, and I always had bladder infections, which made things even worse."

Alicia withdrew as much as she could. "I had no social life. All I wanted to do was sit in my room and read. I felt that I was a bad kid, that I didn't try hard enough. That was what all my teachers told me. I didn't do anything right. It used to make me feel that I was so wrong, that I was some horrible child who couldn't handle life."

Thin as a small child, Alicia started gaining weight. When she was twelve, her parents sent her to a camp designed to help children to lose weight. "That is where I realized that something was very wrong," she says. Activities were scheduled from early morning to lights out at night. Climbing the steep hill to the mess tent, Alicia needed help. Coming down the hill, she invariably fell. "I don't know if it was nutrition or the physical strain on my body, but after the first week I started crying and couldn't stop," she says.

Her parents came to the camp to give her a pep talk. "You're not a quitter. You're a strong person. You can do this," she quotes them. Alicia stayed the whole three weeks, but she came home still crying. "I wasn't eating. I wasn't doing anything. All I could do was cry," she says.

Alicia's parents took her to a psychiatrist. His diagnosis was separation anxiety. He prescribed Xanax, an antianxiety drug. "Separation anxiety was all we talked about. I kept telling him I was so frustrated and confused, but he never asked what I was frustrated and confused about," she says.

Each new school year was the start of another nightmare. "I couldn't sleep. I just kept crying and begging not to have to go to school. At school I was teased, tortured, and stigmatized, even by the teachers. I almost had a nervous breakdown each time I started school," she recalls.

Although she had no right-left dominance, wrote backward, and transposed numbers, Alicia did well academically. "The only thing I ever did poorly in was gym; I always got C's," she says. To this day she has trouble holding a book while reading for lack of strength in her arms and hands. Her parents always asked the school for a spare set of textbooks so that Alicia didn't have to carry her books home and back again.

In fifth grade Alicia failed at an assignment requiring her to memorize the names of the fifty states and their capitals. She speaks of feeling ashamed that she has never been able to name all of the states.

Until she was thirteen, Alicia thought everyone hurt all the time. "I just remember feeling so horrible, but I couldn't share it because I thought that everyone felt the same way, so why should I complain?" she says. Eventually, her parents brought her to a neurologist, who diagnosed her fibromyalgia. "He didn't know very much about it," Alicia recalls. "I remember him saying that it was not degenerative, and that it would not get any worse. He gave me the blue pamphlet that comes from the Arthritis Foundation. I hate that flyer; it makes fibromyalgia sound like a kind of flu and that there's nothing you can do about it."

The neurologist sent Alicia to a rheumatologist. "He handed me a photocopy of the Canadian Air Force exercise book and told me to pick out whatever exercises I could do. Then he told me that I was going to have to learn to live with it," she says. The rheumatologist prescribed Naprosyn, a nonsteroidal anti-inflammatory drug. Before long, Alicia had a stomach ulcer. She has never been able to tolerate any of the medications she tried. "To this day, I still don't take pills," she says.

Once she had a name for her problem, Alicia says she went through all the emotions associated with grieving. "I was angry. I was depressed. I wanted to crawl into a hole and die. I never thought about suicide, but I wondered how anyone so young as I was could deal with all this pain. Everybody thought that by giving it a name it would make things better, but in a way it made everything worse. I wasn't able to pretend anymore that I was normal. But," she adds, "I had an excuse to get out of gym class."

As Alicia grew, she adjusted. By her sophomore year in college, she says, "I had some of the most wonderful friends in the world, and my confidence had increased to the point where I felt I could do anything." Then came a severe flare-up, and Alicia came to the realization that she "could never hold a normal type-A-personality kind of career. It wouldn't be fair to my body. Maybe I could do it if I wanted to live on pills my whole life, but I didn't want that."

Alicia takes a philosophical view of her disorder. "I'm kind of happy that I got it as a child, because I grew up trying harder," she says. A woman at a support group meeting once challenged Alicia, saying, "You have no idea what I'm going through." "I said, 'You're right, because I don't feel that anything was taken away from me. I was born like this. I don't remember going out to play and not feeling pain."

Her big fear these days concerns having children. "The only thing I'm scared about is that people say fibromyalgia is genetic.

In a couple of years I'm going to be having kids, and I don't want them to have to go through what I went through."

Asked if she had advice for children with FM, she says, "There is a great deal you can do, so there's no point in sitting there and being upset about it. Children have the greatest imaginations, and it's very easy to escape if you really try."

CHAPTER EIGHT

FM and Your Private Life

FIBROMYALGIA does not exist in a vacuum. It is part of your life, and you are part of the lives of many other people—parents, a spouse or committed partner, children, neighbors, friends, colleagues, and co-workers. To a greater or lesser degree then, fibromyalgia is part of their lives, too. People close to you and even those in your circle of acquaintances who don't know you have FM may experience its effects on your actions and moods and your ability or inability to live up to their expectations and meet their needs. You need to gain their understanding and support to the extent that is possible. Most of all, you need to protect yourself from a lack of knowledge and insensitivity on the part of those with whom you interact, regardless of the depth or frequency of that interaction.

Spouses and Significant Others

Sad to say, fibromyalgia has played a role in the breakup of many committed relationships. In some cases, it was the last straw in a relationship already strained nearly to the breaking point, but in other instances the fracture could have been prevented if the partners had more knowledge of the disorder and more skill in talking things over. The situation is most perilous in cases where the two people involved were both healthy when they decided to blend their lives. Now that one has fibromyalgia, a great many things must change.

Pat and Chris met on a singles club outing. They soon discovered that they shared a love of nature, being outdoors, and hiking and backpacking. Chris was not as well coordinated as Pat and grew tired more easily, and sometimes Pat's gentle teasing caused a bit of friction, but the two had so much in common that the annoyance seemed minor. Before long they decided that they wanted to be together more often than on weekends. They exchanged vows, moved in together, and announced to the world that they were a couple.

Two years later, Chris was in an automobile accident that resulted in severe back pain. Unable to sleep well, Chris seemed not to be recovering from the accident's effects. As days turned into weeks and weeks into months, Chris spent more and more of the couple's leisure time in bed. Pat longed for the good old days on the hiking trail, but Chris had too much pain and too little energy to muster any enthusiasm for the outdoor activities that had brought them together. Pat felt guilty about wanting to go hiking alone, but eventually went anyway. Chris felt resentful that Pat wanted to go solo, but tried to be a good sport about it. Gradually the two, who had once been the closest of friends and the best of playmates, grew farther and farther apart.

On one level, there is no solution to this kind of problem. Chris can't be expected to go backpacking with pain and fatigue. Pat can't be expected to give up the outdoors because Chris must. Chris has a right to feel frustrated, angry, and left out of the fun. Pat has a right to feel let down, too. If they can't find a way to resolve their negative feelings, the couple is headed for disaster.

The Relationship Contract

Committed relationships are based on a sort of unwritten contract, which defines what the relationship will consist of and what roles the members will play. In the prototypical example of the nuclear family, the man will be the major breadwinner and will assume responsibility for car and home maintenance.

The woman may go out to work, too, but she has primary responsibility for care of the children, or the meals, laundry, and tidiness of the home. The particulars vary from couple to couple, but some kind of unspoken contract exists in every long-term relationship. When one of the parties to the contract becomes ill, roles change. The healthy partner must take on the major share of responsibilities for which he or she may not feel equipped. One husband of a fibromyalgic said this:

> I am employed, but it feels as if I am a single parent. I must now contribute much more to the family than before. While I believe I shared responsibility to the family unit before the condition flared up, I am now having to do so much more, including cooking, cleaning, dishes, laundry, car maintenance, yard work, helping children with homework, carpool driving for children, and of course, a full-time job.

Without thinking about it, most couples include in this unspoken contract the expectation that the significant other will remain in the same state of health as she or he was in when the relationship began. That's where we get into trouble. People with fibromyalgia often look perfectly healthy. Our partners may find it hard to believe that we can't do the things we say we can't do. Many of us are reluctant to talk about our pain. By keeping our feelings to ourselves, we distance ourselves from the people who should be closest to us. Doctors sometimes play a role in the misunderstanding between partners. If the doctor takes an "it's all in your head" attitude toward the person with FM, who can blame an overworked spouse for feeling aggrieved?

If it makes sense to you that part of the problem in a troubled relationship is that the member who has FMS isn't living up to the contract with its assumptions about roles and responsibilities, then anger on the part of the well spouse is an understandable response, as is guilt and/or defensiveness on the part of the person with fibromyalgia. It doesn't matter that neither the anger nor the guilt and defensiveness can be rationally justified. People can't be blamed for the way they feel. Feelings are facts that must be dealt with, by both parties.

If this sounds familiar to you, it may be a good idea to start a conversation on the subject, sometime when interruptions are unlikely and things aren't too tense for a calm appraisal of the situation. Assuming you are the one with FM, you might open the conversation with an honest expression of regret that you can't do all the things you used to be able to do, an expression of hope that the day will come when you're able again, and a promise to learn everything you can about FM to make that day come as soon as possible. Make it possible for your partner to express feelings of anger, fear, or frustration, without having to worry that you will feel attacked and criticized. Acknowledge that for the time being at least, you've each lost something of value in the relationship, and promise to help each other retrieve it.

Grief and Acceptance

Another way to look at the situation is in terms of the grief cycle described by Elizabeth Kübler Ross, in her classic work *On Death and Dying.* She describes the stages that people go through when faced with loss—any significant loss. The stages are shock, denial, rage, bargaining, and acceptance. Each stage may last for a short or a long time. They don't always occur in the same order. You may be in one stage and your partner in another. Either or both of you may repeat some stages and possibly skip, or zoom through, others. Sometimes people get stuck in a stage and never come to acceptance. An outsider's involvement—a professional counselor or wise and trusted friend—can help one or both partners to get unstuck. If you can work this through together, that's wonderful. If you can't, it's not a failure, and you are to be admired and respected for being big enough to admit that you need help.

For the person who has FM, being diagnosed often gives rise to truly ambivalent feelings: dismay that something is wrong that can't be set right, and relief that someone has at long last recognized that something is truly wrong. No matter how empathic the well partner may be, adjustments and accommodations will have to be made. Once the person with FM adjusts to the reality of the disorder, the desire to learn about it, talk about it, go to support groups, and meet others who have it can be exhilarating. The healthy partner has nothing comparable to make up for the loss of a formerly healthy companion. Anger may quickly replace shock—anger at having to assume so many new responsibilities, anger at losing a playmate, anger at the mate's self-absorption in the process of learning about fibromyalgia, anger even at the mate's new friends, with whom there is a bond of shared, painful experience.

I've talked with many people with fibromyalgia whose mates refuse to accompany them to support group meetings, and who even refuse to read a single article on the subject. These mates are in denial. They may feel that if they ignore the situation it will resolve itself—that the person with FM will miraculously get well, or at least stop complaining and resume normal activities. Denial may be a safe refuge for people disappointed at the hand life has dealt, but the issue will have to be faced. Some healthy partners honestly believe that talking about FM will only make the other person feel worse. It's hard to find the balance between talking about it all the time and never discussing it. The two of you will need to do some negotiating to find the proper mixture of discussing all the implications of having a chronic, painful disorder. But it can be done, and for the sake of your relationship, it must be done.

Some healthy mates move into the bargaining stage with a determination to fix the problem. This is a healthy impulse if it's not carried to extremes. Such people plow into research with a vengeance. They may come home from work every day with a new idea for you to try, and they may become infuriated if you don't immediately agree to try it. Or you may try it but find that it doesn't help you. You need to make it clear that people experience fibromyalgia in a variety of ways, and there is as yet no one remedy that helps everyone.

Many people, particularly men, feel responsible for solving the problem and frustrated that they can't. It's easy to imagine how conflict can arise if the healthy partner comes up with solutions that the person with FM declines to try, or tries and reports no improvement.

What it all comes down to is a case of conflicting needs. If you're both feeling needy, and neither one of you is focused on giving, friction is inevitable. Couples who are successful at avoiding strife at such times have learned to do a quick round of negotiation when both partners are in need of sympathy and reassurance. It takes practice, but you can learn to decide whose needs are the greater at the moment and focus on that person, with the understanding that the other's turn will come shortly. To make this work, you must both want it to work, and you must each trust the other to be fair in assessing whose needs get tended to first.

Here are some suggestions that people have offered.

• Learn together, if possible. Knowledge is power, and the more you know about fibromyalgia the more power you will have to control it. Go to support group meetings together and talk about what you heard when you get home. Read everything you can get your hands on. Some articles will contradict others, which is natural in a condition about which so little is known. Finding contradictions gives you the opportunity to talk about your own experience with FM without sounding like you are complaining. Everything you learn will bring you closer together.

• Recognize and affirm each other's feelings. It's hard to hear your spouse complain about having to do so much of the housework, when you'd love to feel well enough to do it yourself, but it's important to listen uncritically, without feeling compelled to defend yourself.

• Put the emphasis on what you *can* do rather than on what you *cannot*. Try to get some spontaneity back into your relationship. If you can't make elaborate plans for a vacation, be flexible enough to suggest an outing or something fun to do on a day when you're feeling comparatively well.

• Find a way to talk about how you feel physically in a neutral, uncomplaining manner. For example, you might agree on a feeling scale of one to ten, with one being terrible and ten being the best you've ever felt. Then, if your partner asks you to do something that you don't feel up to, you might say, "I'm at about five today. When I hit seven, I'll be glad to."

• Find a way to explain the pain so that your partner can understand. One man said he couldn't understand what FM pain was like until he was asked to remember how he felt after several consecutive all-nighters at finals time in college.

• Find a way to handle what seem like dismissive remarks. Among fibromyalgics the term "brain fog" is understood, but if you try to explain it to someone who does not have FM, the person is likely to reply, "But I forget people's names, too, and sometimes I have trouble finding the car keys." Assume that this is meant to make you feel better and observe—gently, if possible—that since the person knows what an occasional lapse feels like, that should make it easier to understand what it's like to be that way all the time.

• If your partner says something that hurts, say so, but do it in a constructive spirit. Unless you have good reason to know otherwise, you should assume that your partner is your best friend and would not willingly say or do anything to hurt you. Say what you think you heard and how those words made you feel, but do it in a questioning way so that your partner can explain what was really meant.

• Approach working through your adjustment to FM in a spirit of optimism and goodwill. Something drew you together. Try to remember and recapture whatever it was. As you learn to communicate about this new factor in your life together, you will come closer to each other. There is joy in that. Let yourself experience it.

Sexual Intimacy

For most people, sex is an important part of a committed relationship. When pain enters the picture, sexual expression can become a problem. In addition, some medications can cause a reduction in sexual desire (libido). If you are experiencing sexual problems of this nature, this section offers some suggestions that may help you.

Many people who have fibromyalgia discover that their interest in sex has diminished. Still others are no less interested, but find sexual activity to be painful, fatiguing, or both. In either case, they are apt to worry about what the loss or lessening of sex will do to their committed relationship. This is a valid concern and one that requires attention.

First it may be helpful to think about what has caused desire to lessen. Pain is an obvious turn-off, but with care and patience it can be minimized. A more subtle cause of loss of libido may be the change in your body image that your FM diagnosis or a period of undiagnosed chronic pain has brought about. The more pride you took in your body—the way it looked, the way it obeyed your directions, and the way it brought you pleasure—the harder it is to accept that it is somewhat less than perfect. This blow to your ego may well translate into a blow to your sexuality.

However, here, as is true in so much of life, what you tell yourself determines how you feel. You can concentrate on the negatives and be miserable, or you can remind yourself of the love you have experienced and that your partner is far less interested in how you look than in who you are. You are not fibromyalgia and fibromyalgia is not you. That you have FM does not make you any less sensual or any less able to give and receive pleasure.

Honest communication between partners is fundamental to the success of any relationship, and it becomes even more vital when illness strikes. If you need reassurance that you are still attractive to your partner, ask for it as clearly as you can so that you will not be misunderstood and disappointed in the response. If certain activities cause you pain, say so and be prepared to discuss alternatives. Talk about what you like and find out what pleases your partner. Challenge your own creativity and that of your partner in discovering new positions and new techniques that take the pressure away from tender places.

Despite the importance of sexual fulfillment to the quality of one's life, few doctors are comfortable discussing the subject during an office visit. There are still too many doctors who think that sex is not important to women, or to elderly people. If you have a doctor you can trust to take your sexual problems seriously, by all means bring up the subject. But if you are not satisfied with the response, don't blame yourself, and don't give up.

Some of the medicines doctors prescribe for FM have a lessening of sexual desire as one of their side effects. Tricyclics do this to some people; Prozac is well known for this effect. If you suspect this is the cause of your lack of interest in sex, you should mention this to your doctor and explore the possibility of trying a different prescription.

Here are general suggestions for keeping fibromyalgia from interfering with intimacy:

• Develop a system of signals that you and your partner can recognize as signs of interest or disinterest in sex.

• Plan to make love at the time of day when you are at your best. It doesn't always have to happen at night.

• If sex is on the agenda, plan an easy day. Avoid activities that will leave you tired and worn-out. But if you feel that way, ask for a raincheck.

• Adjust the time you take your pain medication so that its effect will be at its maximum during sex.

• Take a warm bath or shower before you go to bed to help your muscles to relax. Sharing the bath or shower with your partner can be the beginning of foreplay.

• Try a change of venue. Go to a motel that has a waterbed. The waterbed's rocking motion can make your own motions less strenuous.

• Experiment with less strenuous ways of getting and giving pleasure. Consult books, videos, or sex therapists for advice on positions and alternative methods of sexual satisfaction.

• Be sure your partner knows where your sore spots are and just how little pressure you can tolerate there. It's better to discuss this when you are not engaging in sex and preferably not in the bedroom.

• Try a variety of positions. Books such as Alex Comfort's *The Joy of Sex* can stimulate your imagination.

• Give yourself a background of sensuous, romantic music. Light candles.

• Don't get focused on orgasm as the only goal of sex. Enjoy the closeness and sensual pleasure even if orgasm eludes you. Don't take the lack of an orgasm as a sign of failure.

• Above all, communicate. Talk about what feels good and what does not. Talk about your feelings. Get the reassurance you need, but remember that your partner has feelings and needs reassurance, too.

With two of you working on it together, satisfying sex need not be an insurmountable problem. Honesty, a generous spirit, and a determination to make it work are the ingredients of success.

Explaining FM to Children

Our children know when we're sick even if we don't tell them. Children notice the strain in our faces, the winces when we move. Even the littlest ones pick up our signals like powerful antennae. There's no use pretending that all is well when it isn't.

However, even though your children know when you're feeling poorly, there is a good reason for telling them what's wrong. Children have vivid imaginations. They are also aware of how dependent they are. If you don't level with them, they will probably imagine something far worse than the truth. One woman told how her college-age daughter quoted her younger sister as saying, "I think Mom is dying and they're not telling me." More than one child of a person with FM has assumed the parent has cancer. No child should have to live with such unjustified fear. What you say depends of course on the age of the child. The basic message to small children should be something like, "I have a sickness that makes me hurt a lot of the time, but it's not going to make me be dead."

To decide what to say when, use the rule that many parents use in teaching about reproduction. Children ask questions when they're ready to hear the answers. In the case of FM, you may have to cast some broad hints around, but they'll pick up the fact that something isn't quite right with you anyway, and you need to create the atmosphere in which they can ask questions. Don't hide from them.

If the child wants to play with you, and the game is something you are physically unable to take part in, you might explain that you are extra tired or your shoulder hurts, and suggest an alternative activity that you can do, or ask the child to suggest one.

As children grow older they can understand more about your physical limitations, and you should be as open with them as you can be. This does not mean going into detail about the aches and pains, no matter how old the child is, but it does mean giving clear messages about what you can and cannot do. For example, one mother talked about her inability to wait up for her teenage children when they went out on dates. Her equilibrium depended on going to bed at the same time each night, and as much as she wanted to be awake when her children came home, she could not afford to disrupt her schedule. Teens may complain when their parents wait up for them, but most secretly like it; it makes them feel secure to know that someone cares whether they get home safely and on time. A mother who does not wait up without giving her child an explanation risks appearing to be emotionally distant and indifferent. I know this from firsthand experience.

My children are all independent adults now. I had FM when I was raising them, but they did not know the nature of my illness until a few years ago, when they were all in their thirties. I think now it was a mistake not telling them how poorly I felt at times when they were small, but I was trying to protect them from worrying about me and feeling insecure. I tried to hide my physical problems from them but it was clear that my charade often failed miserably. Since I told them about fibromyalgia, they understand why I was sometimes not available to them as much as they wanted me to be. As a result, they accept the circumstances of their childhood much better now that they know about my FM than they did before, and we have grown even closer and more like friends.

The good side of that is that they often turned to each other for support and are still good friends, although they are geographically dispersed. They also learned to do things around the house that parents usually do—cooking and laundry, for example. They grew up to be competent and self-sufficient.

Your physical problem provides an ideal opportunity to increase your child's understanding of individual differences. You can point out that everyone has different abilities; some people cannot take part in active sports, but they can do other interesting things, such as art, music, or some other activity that you value. You might invite your child to join you in thinking creatively about things you can enjoy together. Above all, be honest and reassuring, but don't try to do things that will cause you further pain and distress.

If you have fibromyalgia there is an increased likelihood that your child will have at least the tendency to develop it. If that child grows up under stress and doesn't feel safe at home—physically and emotionally—that child is almost certain to develop it at some triggering point in her or his life. There are two things you can do to minimize the likelihood that your child will experience fibromyalgia. Neither is guaranteed to avoid it, but the two together maximize the chances that your child will grow up healthier than you are.

First, it is important to strive for a family atmosphere that is as nearly free of stress as possible. Links between FM and stress have been documented. That does not mean that stress causes fibromyalgia, but it has been shown that the adrenal glands in people with FM have a tendency to overreact to stress, making the condition worse.

Second, children who may have a tendency to develop FM later in life should be taught the principles of healthful living while they are still young enough to adopt them as habits.

Children should be taught to appreciate healthful snacks. Food should never be used to punish or reward. The habit of going to bed at the same time each night should begin in early childhood. The value of regular exercise should be taught and demonstrated from the earliest years. Helping your child to develop good health habits is the best thing you can do for the child, whether or not you suspect a predisposition to fibromyalgia.

Explaining FM to Family and Friends

Parents of adult offspring often have difficulty hearing about their children's illness. Some people want to believe that they have raised perfect physical specimens, and fibromyalgia certainly denies them this pleasure. If you think now that you had signs of FM in childhood, it may be tempting to tell your parents so, but you should be prepared to face a wall of denial, behind which lurks guilt.

> Ginny and her seventy-five-year-old father lived on opposite coasts and talked frequently on the telephone. Ginny wanted

to tell her father about her fibromyalgia and the effect it was having on her life, but he kept changing the subject. She wrote a long letter describing her symptoms, telling him she felt as though she had "a bad case of influenza, with jet lag on top of it." Her father wrote back saying he was sorry she didn't feel well and hoped she'd be better soon. "It hurts me that my father can't understand that I am a different person since I developed this condition," Ginny says. "Perhaps it's too over-whelming. Maybe he thinks he should be able to 'fix' me and feels helpless because he can't."

Perhaps Ginny will never be able to gain her father's under-standing. Her conjecture is probably very close to the truth. The problem is especially difficult for fibromyalgics who have unre-solved issues with their parents, particularly if they resent that their parents did not take their childhood complaints of pain seriously. It's almost impossible to conceal feelings of that sort, even if your words carry a different message. Some people find it best to write about their feelings or tell them to a tape re-corder, just to get them off their chest. Then they throw away the writing or erase the tape. Having done that, they are ready to talk to their parents about their experience of FM without rancor.

Telling friends and acquaintances is another matter. Some people tell everyone; others tell no one. To some extent, you need the people around you to understand your condition so that they will understand when you cancel an engagement at the last minute and pull back from outside activities. You may find it difficult to hold up your end of a relationship when your energy is low and your pain is high. You probably look healthy enough; if you don't confide in your friends, they may think you are rejecting them when you cancel engagements or never seem to want to do anything together. The trick is to give people enough detail so that they understand that you still want to be included in their plans, but not so much that they feel over-whelmed. Be sure, by the way, to stress that FM is not life-threatening. You don't want to be the subject of an unjustified death watch—children are not the only people who tend to think the worst if they don't have the facts.

Pregnancy, Childbirth, and Postpartum Care

The burning question for many women of childbearing age is whether they should become pregnant. There is no simple answer to this question, and certainly no answer that will apply to all women. However, there are some factors to take into consideration.

• Many doctors tell fibromyalgics to stop all medications *before* they conceive and most say to stop them as soon as you know you are pregnant. Since it would be unethical to conduct drug testing on pregnant women, almost nothing is known about the effects of drugs on an embryo (the fertilized egg up to the end of the eighth week after conception) or fetus. If you are considering pregnancy or are already pregnant, discuss with your doctor every drug you are taking, whether by prescription or over the counter.

• Before you become pregnant, get yourself into the best possible physical condition. Pregnancy and childbirth are strenuous; raising a child is, too. Do whatever you can to improve your strength and muscle tone, particularly in your back and abdominal muscles. Think more than twice about getting pregnant if you can't do any form of exercise.

• Many women find that their symptoms decrease or even disappear during pregnancy. It may be that the extra amounts of female hormones present during pregnancy cause muscles and ligaments to relax, relieving pain.

• Many drugs used to treat FM find their way into breast milk. If you plan on nursing, you must take this into account.

• Plan to have help for a few weeks after delivery, especially during the night. If you are bottle-feeding, ask your husband to handle the nighttime duties. If you are nursing, ask your husband to bring the baby to you, change the diapers, and put the baby back in the crib so that your sleep will be minimally disturbed. Learn to express breast milk into nursing bottles and refrigerate or freeze them so you won't have to be awakened when someone else cares for the baby during the night. This will help you to maintain your milk supply even though you are not personally involved in nighttime feedings. You will be especially vulnerable to FM flare-up after you deliver, and having your sleep disturbed will surely make things worse.

• Consider taking a high-dose, yeast-free B-complex tablet (50 or 100 mg per day) for at least a month after the baby is born. The female hormone estrogen consumes large quantities of B vitamins; this is thought by many to be the cause of the postpartum depression that strikes many mothers about three weeks after delivery. B-vitamin deficiency can also cause joint and nerve pains.

CASE HISTORY: THE BROWN FAMILY

Natalie Brown, a forty-four-year-old teacher, is the only one in her family who does not have fibromyalgia. Her husband David, a photographer, also forty-four, realizes now that he has probably had FM since he was eight years old. Their son, Jonathan, eleven, started having symptoms when he was eight, and was diagnosed at ten. Daughter, Janice, thirteen, recently got her FM diagnosis as well. "It has been a difficult journey," Natalie says. "The fact that the medical community is not really on top of FM, especially in children, was frustrating for all of us."

David recalls having stomach pains as a child. "The doctor couldn't find anything wrong and said I had a 'tight stomach.' He gave me some sort of stomach-relaxing medication, and the pain went away after a few months," he says. Soon after that, he started having trouble with his knee. "Until I was in my twenties, it would give me pain every few months. The doctor said I probably had a cracked cartilage, but as long as the pain was in the upper knee, he said not to worry about it."

His parents gave him swimming lessons when he was very young, and by the time he was five David was a competitive swimmer. He thinks now that swimming protected him from serious FM bouts in childhood. When the swim team broke up when he was thirteen, David tried skiing and tennis. "I never did well in team sports," he remarks.

During his teens and twenties, David had episodes of unexplained pain, but it took an auto accident when he was thirty-six, in which he injured his neck, to bring his fibromyalgia to the forefront. He wore a neck brace for nine months, then started physical therapy. "I would get to a point where things were going well. Then the physical therapist would give me a one-pound weight to exercise with and it would set me back to the way I was on day one," he says. A neurologist did nerve-conduction tests; they were all normal. The neurologist had just read an article about fibrositis, as FM used to be called, and suggested that David see a rheumatologist and find out if that was what he had.

The rheumatologist confirmed that David had FM and prescribed a muscle relaxant and an NSAID for pain. Three weeks later, after nine months of undiagnosed suffering, David was back at work full time. He remained relatively symptom-free for the next three years.

During that time, Jonathan, who was then eight, started having strange symptoms—stomachaches, bladder spasms, and random unexplained pain. "No one made the connection between what was going on with Jonathan and what my husband had," Natalie says. Within a matter of months, David developed stomach problems, probably caused by the NSAIDs, that eventually led to surgery. Within the same year, he also had two spinal operations related to his neck injury. "I think after a while you become numb," Natalie says. "I had to deal with the hospital,

David's recovery, Jonathan's pain, and not knowing what was wrong with him. The only way I could do that was just to put one foot in front of the other and go on to the next step."

A series of doctors put Jonathan through a series of tests— "cystoscopies, MRIs, CAT scans, bone scans, and much blood work," Natalie says. "I knew the pain he was in. I held him nightly while he cried and screamed as he urinated or had tremendous back pain." The succession of doctors suggested psychological testing, or a summer at camp. One asked "if there might be a daycare worker that had abused Jonathan," Natalie adds.

Determined to find help for her son, in the summer of 1994 Natalie took Jonathan to the Mayo Clinic, where a doctor did a tender point exam, diagnosed fibromyalgia, and told her they "had nothing to offer other than what we were doing." Natalie started doing her own research. She found a paper by Abraham Gedalia, M.D., on FM in children, and arranged to have him see Jonathan, who was at this point in such pain that he was confined to a wheelchair.

Natalie needed time off to take Jonathan to see Dr. Gedalia, but the school system where she taught would not pay for a leave of absence unless she herself was ill. "The only way I could get paid my salary and have money for the trip, was to declare myself mentally incapable of doing my job. I went to my doctor and asked him for a note saying that I needed a leave of absence. That's how I was able to take a month off to deal with Jonathan's problems," she says.

Dr. Gedalia admitted Jonathan to a children's hospital for a week of physical therapy. By the end of the week, Jonathan was walking again.

Jonathan's relief from pain lasted only a few weeks, however. Continuing her research, Natalie found the fibromyalgia discussion group on the Internet, where she learned about Paul St. Amand, M.D., and his guaifenesin treatment (see chapter six). "We put Jonathan on guaifenesin in May 1995, and have watched the process unfold," she says. "Within the first four days, Jonathan started to have pains in his knees and ankles. We were encouraged, as this is what it [guaifenesin] is supposed to do. This episode lasted about two weeks and then overnight the pain was gone. We were elated."

Other symptoms followed, and the Browns decided it was time to take Jonathan to see Dr. St. Amand, a thousand-mile trip. The whole family went. Dr. St. Amand examined Jonathan and David and charted their areas of pain. Janice asked to be examined as well, and was also diagnosed with FM. "We were really surprised about that, but now after thinking about it we realize she had signs along the way."

David, Janice, and Jonathan are all taking guaifenesin now, and all are showing signs of improvement. Jonathan is out of his wheelchair and riding his bike with friends after school.

Natalie admits that Jonathan and more recently Janice are the focus of her energies. Of David, she says, "He pretty much manages for himself. My way of dealing with all this is to detach myself from his problems, but I can't detach myself from my children's problems. It's a protection not to get too emotionally involved with every ache and pain that David has. Instead of getting angry and upset that he can't help me clean the house, although there were many times when it did upset me, I just put up a little wall between his problems and what I need to do."

Natalie hopes the resulting strain on her marriage is a temporary thing. "Intimacy has really been a secondary part of our life for a long time," she says. "I've learned to say it's not a big deal to me. We probably could use time to nurture each other and develop a stronger relationship, but right now we're just trying to see where this leads. Hopefully, if we ever get to the end of it, things will be better for all of us."

CHAPTER NINE

Fibromyalgia and Work

WORK is a necessity for people with fibromyalgia just as it is for most everyone else. But working with FM presents special challenges. Even a desk job can be physically difficult. Most people who have fibromyalgia stiffen up about the hips and knees if they have been sitting for any length of time. They need to be able to get up and move about every thirty minutes or so. People who have their hands on a keyboard for hours on end suffer from pain in the hands, wrists, elbows, and shoulders. They need a workstation that is designed to conform to the principles of ergonomics, the applied science of arranging the things people use in their work for maximum comfort, safety, and efficiency. Office workers are often expected to lift cartons of files and office supplies, but lifting an object that weighs as little as ten pounds is often beyond the capabilities of a person with FM.

I know of a woman employed as a secretary who was threatened with dismissal when she told her supervisor she was unable to climb two flights of stairs to wash out a coffeepot. The woman had never mentioned fibromyalgia to her supervisor, who saw the secretary's refusal to wash a coffeepot as insubordination.

Another woman lost her administrative job when she scheduled a meeting for October that was supposed to be held in September, and canceled another meeting on her boss's instructions, but forgot to notify the people coming from all over the country to attend it that it had been canceled.

The cognitive difficulties that often accompany FM pose a major problem for those who are classified as "knowledge workers." A university professor told me, "I used to be a real star, and now I can't do anything. This is so hard to accept. My memory is fading away and I get paid for thinking. All I've ever had going for me was my IQ and now I just watch it slip away from me. What will be left if I don't have the use of my faculties of reason and understanding?"

Not every fibromyalgia-caused work problem can be solved by asking for accommodation or assistance, but some can be. Because of widespread ignorance about fibromyalgia, people who have it are not as likely to be excused from painful tasks, or given adaptive devices to help them work, as are people with rheumatoid arthritis (RA). Yet a 1989 study that compared 116 people with FM with 106 who had rheumatoid arthritis found that one-third of those who had FM had to change jobs at least once because of their condition, compared with one-fourth of those with RA.

To Tell or Not to Tell

Of course, asking for help or special dispensation at work means telling your supervisor, and perhaps your co-workers. There are arguments for and against disclosing your condition at work.

Here are the arguments for disclosure.

• Disclosure gives you the right to ask for reasonable accommodations under terms of the Americans with Disabilities Act (about which you will read more later in this chapter).

• If there is a chance that you will ever need to file a complaint on grounds of harassment or discrimination based on disability, there must be a record of your problem. You can't complain that the company refused to accommodate your needs if your employer doesn't know of those needs.

• If there is a chance you will ever need to file for short- or long-term disability, the fact that you have FM must appear on your record at work.

• Perhaps most significantly, being open about your condition relieves you of the need to spend energy on appearing to feel well and energetic when you do not.

The arguments against disclosure are these.

• If you change jobs, the fact that you have fibromyalgia might cause a new insurance company to rule that anything that sends you to a doctor is a preexisting condition. There is some limit under U.S. law to the insurance company's right to deny you insurance coverage, however.

• Some people experience discrimination in the form of harassment or lack of promotion opportunities if they report a chronic illness.

• Co-workers may distance themselves because they feel uncomfortable and don't know how to treat a person who is chronically unwell.

One woman told me that she makes disclosure her policy whenever she interviews for a job. She explains her condition, acknowledges that she is not sure that she will always be able to work full time, or even part time, and promises to keep her employer as informed as she is about the state of her health. She believes she has never lost a job opportunity on the basis of her physical condition.

Another told her superiors when she started in a new position that she had trouble with her knees, but not about her fibromyalgia. "Now that I am in the midst of a major flare-up, I find myself having to explain why I have had trouble maintaining my schedule recently. Looking back, I think it might have been easier if I had at least spoken to my department head after I started working here," she says.

Your instincts will tell you whether you are working for the kind of employer who can handle the knowledge of your fibromyalgia intelligently and sensitively. If you tell people you have fibromyalgia, you need to be prepared with a brief and clear description that will make sense to them. You might try something like this: Fibromyalgia is a disorder that causes pain, problems with sleeping, and sometimes severe fatigue. Its cause and cure are not known, but it is not life-threatening or contagious.

As a writer, I work for myself, which means that every editor who gives me an assignment is my boss on that project. You can be sure that I leave out any mention of cognitive dysfunction if I tell an editor about fibromyalgia at all—and, until I started writing this book, I didn't tell any of them. I don't talk about flare-ups either, because no editor needs to stay awake worrying about whether I will get my article in on time. My clients can't see me work, so they don't know if I take a day off during the week and work on a weekend instead, and they don't care. All they care about is that I get my work in by deadline, and I always do.

If you are likely to need accommodations at work, such as a special chair or being relieved of certain duties, you will probably find it beneficial to tell your co-workers what the problem is. There may be some who are envious of any perceived "special treatment," refuse to believe you, or think you are trying to find a way to get out of doing your work, but for the most part you will probably find that people's reactions range from neutral to sympathetic. You can help cement good relationships with co-workers who are required to do some of the work you cannot do by offering to do some of their work. If people see you are willing to do as much as you can, they are less likely to discredit and discount your condition.

The Americans with Disabilities Act

If you live in the United States and are having trouble performing all the duties required of you at work, the Americans with

Disabilities Act (ADA) may furnish you with needed help and protection. Among many other provisions, it requires employers to make reasonable accommodations for employees with disabilities.

You do not have to be disabled in the sense of qualifying for disability payments to have a disability. The law defines disability as a physical or mental impairment that substantially limits one or more of your major life activities. If fibromyalgia prevents you from lifting anything heavier than ten pounds, you have a disability as far as lifting is concerned. You meet the law's definition of a "qualified individual with a disability" if you are capable of performing the essential functions of your job or the job for which you are applying with or without reasonable accommodations. In case of a dispute, the law takes into consideration the employer's judgment as to what functions of the job are essential. If there is a written job description, that defines the job's essential functions. According to the ADA, functions other than those that are essential to the job must be modified or transferred to another employee. Bear in mind that the catchall phrase included in many job descriptions "and other duties as required" does not meet the ADA criteria for essential functions.

Reasonable accommodations include making existing facilities readily accessible to and usable by individuals with disabilities, as well as job restructuring, part-time or modified work schedules, acquisition or modification of equipment or devices, the provision of qualified readers or interpreters, and several other similar accommodations. (See Appendix A for sources of more information on the Americans with Disabilities Act.)

There are two exceptions to these provisions. First is that they don't apply in a company that has fewer than fifteen employees—that is, people working for the entire company, not just in your department or location—unless the company has voluntarily adopted the law. Also, an exception can be made if the accommodation would cause an undue hardship on your employer. Undue hardships are generally considered to be significant difficulty or expense, determined by the nature and cost of the accommodation required and the financial resources of the company.

Thus, if you have severe low back pain and require an adjustable chair with a lumbar support, you have a legitimate right to ask your employer to provide one. Some people whose jobs require a significant amount of keyboarding have been provided with voice-activated computer software so that they no longer have to type at all. Some people who have fibromyalgia have been excused from otherwise mandatory overtime work because the extra effort puts them at risk of a flare-up. There are many accommodations that are relatively inexpensive but make it possible for people with FM to work productively where they otherwise could not.

If you ask your employer for an accommodation, you are most likely to be successful if you offer a solution rather than just state your problem. The more information you can provide about your solution—including, if possible, suppliers and costs—the more likely you are to succeed in getting what you need. A calm, constructive approach always works best, but keep in mind that the law specifically prohibits any retaliation, coercion, or intimidation of a person who makes a request for accommodation under the ADA, or any interference with the person's exercise of rights under this law. You cannot be fired for having FM, asking for relief from tasks that are difficult or painful for you, or for requesting equipment that will help you do your job, and you also cannot be punished for asking for accommodations under the law.

Remedies are spelled out in the law for people who feel they have not been treated properly, but some of them cost money and involve going to court. If you do sue and win, you can have your legal fees paid by the losing party, but in practice you will probably decide that legal action is not worth the energy and stress it will cost you. If you make what seems to you a reasonable request and that request is denied, there are agencies and organizations that may help, but their backlogs are often extensive, so it's worth preparing your request and planning your approach carefully before you begin.

Office Ergonomics

Good posture is especially important when you have FM. The basic principle of office ergonomics is that everything at your workstation, including the position of your back, legs, and arms should be either vertical or horizontal.

- The back of the chair should support you in an upright position, with support for your lower back.
- The computer monitor and copy holder should be at eye level.
- Your forearms and upper thighs should be parallel to the floor.
- Your wrists should be in a straight line with your forearms when your hands are on the keyboard.
- Your feet should be flat on the floor, or on a footrest.

If you feel pain across the tops of your shoulders, your keyboard is too high; raise your chair seat. If your legs ache, your chair is too high; either lower it or get a footrest to raise your feet. A telephone book or two can be used in an emergency until your employer provides the needed footrest.

Few employers realize this, but your chair is probably the single most important piece of equipment in your office. This would be true if you did not have FM, but it is especially true when you do. A good chair is adjustable as to the height of the seat, and the height of the back. It should be wide enough to accommodate your hips. The seat should be adjustable so that it does not cause pressure on the underside of your thighs. If it is a rolling chair, it should have five feet, not four.

Your computer monitor and office lighting should be arranged so that you do not see reflections on the monitor screen. You may find that you have fewer headaches if you make this simple adjustment. Office and computer supply stores carry filters that attach to the monitor to block glare, a good solution if rearranging the office is not possible.

Working at Home

Perhaps you can't go to a job the way you once could. Maybe you have too much pain, or took off too many sick days and were let go. After you've done your grieving, think about something you can do to contribute to society and get something back, such as money and self-respect.

If you're out of a job, or nearly so, it helps to think about getting *work* as opposed to getting another job. Instead of having one employer who has the power to fire you, having several clients really provides more security. It's easier to find a new customer than a new boss.

One way to go into business for yourself is to think of all the things you'd pay someone to do for you, then pick one or two and offer to do them for other people.

The only way I know of to *stay* in business is to give your customers a little more and a little better than they expected. When they praise you, remind them that you do this for your living and you'd appreciate it if they will tell their friends about you. It should go without saying that you must be *absolutely reliable*.

That sounds like a conflict with FM, I know, but it doesn't have to be that way. I've been in the business of writing magazine articles and books since 1983 and I've always given myself long lead times. From the beginning, when it was a lie, I told editors that I was usually booked six weeks in advance, so they shouldn't count on me for emergency last-minute assignments, but were always free to ask. They got the idea early on that I was much in demand, and that made me all the more attractive as a writer. It also gave (and gives) me time to have bad days and still not miss a deadline. I've been plenty sick and laid up at times during these years, but I still haven't missed a deadline. (Twice I've hired other writers to help me out, sharing a byline and fee with them, but that's as bad as it's gotten.)

A good job for people who have fibromyalgia, I think, is something you can do largely at home, that allows you to negotiate long lead times, and that doesn't involve a lot of stress or performance pressure.

Many people, particularly if they are disabled or depressed, underestimate their abilities and can't imagine what they might have to offer that others would want to pay for. On one of your better days, list all the jobs you have held, whether for pay or as a volunteer, and all the skills involved in performing those jobs. If you have raised a family, be sure to include that as one of your jobs, and think of all the organizing, financial management, administrative, nurturing, and leadership skills involved. Turn off that tape running in the back of your mind that says, "You can't do that." No matter how much you have lost, there are still plenty of things you can do. Try. Take chances. You'll surprise yourself, and enrich your life and the lives of others as well.

Filing a Disability Claim

According to the American Association of Disabled Persons, 48.9 million Americans, or more than 19 percent of the total U.S. population, have some type of disability. Of these, 24.1 million, or nearly 10 percent of the total population, have a severe disability. Back or spinal problems account for 3.9 million disabilities, arthritis or rheumatism another 2.7 million. About 8 million disabled people under age sixty-five receive government disability insurance payments. This section is about applying for Social Security disability benefits, but it is not intended to provide legal advice. For that you may want to consult a lawyer who specializes in disability issues. The National Organization of Social Security Claims Representatives (800-431-2804) refers people to private attorneys specializing in Social Security claims law.

You do not necessarily need a lawyer to file your claim, but you will almost certainly be turned down the first time and may well want a lawyer to represent you after that. Typically, a Social Security disability lawyer will charge you 25 percent of the

amount you receive when your claim is approved. That amount
should be calculated as of the day you first became disabled.

It is important to understand the Social Security Administration's idea of what it means to be disabled. This is the U.S.
government's definition of disability:

> The inability to engage in any substantial gainful activity by
> reason of any medically determinable physical or mental im-
> pairment, which can be expected to result in death or which
> has lasted or can be expected to last for a continuous period of
> not less than twelve months. A person must not only be unable
> to do his or her previous work but also cannot, considering age,
> education, and work experience, engage in any other kind of
> substantial gainful work that exists in the national economy. It
> is immaterial whether such work exists in the immediate area,
> or whether a specific job vacancy exists, or whether the worker
> would be hired if he or she applied for work.

Qualifying for disability under this definition may sound like
quite a mountain to climb, but keep this in mind: If you can't
hold anything in your hand for more than five minutes at a time,
you can't qualify for a job that requires you to write by hand. If
you can't stand up for more than fifteen minutes at a time, you
can't qualify for a job that requires you to work on your feet.
Thus, you have just been disqualified for the most common
"substantial gainful activity," flipping burgers at the local fast-
food chain. If you can't sit for more than twenty minutes at a
time, you can't qualify for any office job. Knowing this may make
qualifying for disability pay seem more possible.

If you are fairly sure you will eventually apply for Social Security disability, think hard about cutting back on your work hours
before you finally leave work altogether, because your monthly
award, when you finally prevail, will be based on your most recent earnings. One fibromyalgic said, "My employer was wonderful about accommodating my difficulties in working. I went
from sixty to forty to twenty to ten hours a week, and I still
couldn't cope, which is probably the reason that my application
was approved the first time. But my working hours decreased

quite rapidly. If I had worked part time for a few years, I would have seriously diminished what Social Security pays me."

The process starts when you file a claim at your local Social Security Administration district office in person. You may also start the process with a telephone call (800-772-1213). You will be asked the nature of your disability, your doctor's name, address, and phone number, and the details of your last job. The SSA will then perform an investigation of your medical history, including your capacity for lifting, walking, sitting, and standing and your work history, citizenship, and insurance coverage. This investigation can take as long as eight months.

Your initial application will almost certainly be denied. If you expect this, you are less likely to be upset when the denial arrives in the mail. You have sixty days from the date the notice was mailed in which to file an appeal, called a "request for reconsideration." Don't wait to appeal. There is nothing to be gained by waiting, and impending cuts in the federal budget will probably stretch the process out longer than what is described here. Every day you wait to appeal may mean two or more additional days of delay in getting your case considered.

You may handle this first appeal yourself, or you may decide that this is the right time to engage an attorney. The appeal triggers the start of a more thorough investigation, which will probably include an examination by an SSA physician, who typically knows nothing about fibromyalgia and is more interested in pleasing the agency by rejecting your claim than in helping you. Be prepared for this phase to last at least six months and to end in a second rejection.

Now you have another sixty days to file a "request for hearing." This is a trial before an administrative law judge; it is usually held within four months. If you have been working alone until now, it is time to bring in an attorney. You will be called on to testify, and so will your physician. If the judge decides against you, you have another sixty days to appeal to the appeals council. Their decision, which will come usually within eight months, will probably agree with the judge. Your move at this point is to file suit in the U.S. district court that serves your hometown. You must be represented in district court by an attorney admitted to practice there. If the district court judge disagrees with the previous decisions denying you disability benefits, the case will probably be remanded (sent back for a new hearing). Since a district court judge has now indicated disagreement with the original denial, your chances of getting a favorable decision are much improved.

This discouraging scenario presents the worst you can expect. My purpose in painting such a glum picture is not to discourage you from applying for assistance. Rather, I want you to be prepared for a long process so that you do not get depressed by what is likely to be a long string of disapprovals and delays. Half of the people who file for disability payments get discouraged and give up after the first or second denial. "I firmly believe that they do this on purpose," says one disability applicant whose case is heading for the appeals council. "They drag it out as long as possible, figuring that by the time your hearing comes you'll either have given up in frustration or will be well enough that you no longer qualify."

You are not helpless. There are things you can do to improve your chances of a favorable decision at an early stage in the process. From the moment you decide that filing for disability is inevitable, keep a daily diary of how you feel and the things you cannot do or have difficulty in doing. Don't overlook anything: the pain you have when getting out of bed, the cramps in your fingers after holding a pen for five minutes, the way your pain medications make you sleepy, your brain fog and inability to remember things. If you can't write, use a tape recorder, remembering to say the date and time each time you record a note, and have someone transcribe the tapes.

Enlist your doctor's support. Every office visit should include a report from you, or a test by the doctor, of your diminished ability to perform the basic functions for useful work—lifting, carrying, standing, walking, sitting—problems with concentration and memory, problems with medication, and anything else that may be pertinent. The SSA decision makers will be looking for as much objective data as possible—lab tests, performance tests, and tests measuring pain levels using an instrument known as a dolorimeter are more persuasive than your reports of pain, fatigue, and so forth. You should also provide evidence of your psychosocial and adaptive behavior, including the ability to interact appropriately with others, to follow instructions, and to keep to a regular schedule. Unfortunately, the harder you try to make the best of your condition, the less likely you are to obtain disability assistance.

Your doctor should be familiar with the Social Security Administration's medical evaluation criteria, found in the "Listing of Impairments" (or just the "Listing") that is contained in the handbook "Disability Evaluation Under Social Security." You can obtain a copy by writing to the Office of Medical Evaluation of the Office of Disability, SSA, 6401 Security Boulevard, Baltimore, MD 21235. Ask for SSA publication No. 64-039.

So far, there is no specific listing for fibromyalgia, so people often use other categories. Don't let your pride get in the way of accepting a diagnosis that the Social Security people will understand, even if it has psychiatric connotations.

This chapter has, I hope, given you many things to think about. I hope you have found help here in keeping your job or if working is no longer possible for you, I hope you will find the techniques and strength to follow through on applying for disability assistance. There is no disgrace involved in taking advantage of a program that the citizens of this country have endorsed and for which you have paid taxes.

To close on a positive note, read the words of a woman who received disability approval on her first try.

> In a nutshell, document everything. Keep going to the doctor. Don't be afraid of a psychiatric exam; it actually helps. Details of the loss of your ability to carry out normal activities of daily living are more important than vague complaints such as "I can't work." Note how things like grooming, driving, shopping, cooking, eating, and cleaning are affected by the disorder, compared with the way you used to do them. Include items such as care of children, social events, and hobbies. Always compare then versus now, saying which you can no longer do and being specific about why.

Many of us tend to minimize our problems when talking with others who don't have FM. We've had too much negative feedback and hesitate to complain. Social Security needs to hear the reality of how your condition affects your life.

CASE HISTORY: MELINDA, 46, DIRECTOR OF
COMPUTER OPERATIONS

Melinda has a very technical and responsible job overseeing computer operations at a large teaching hospital. She received her diagnosis in 1992, after a year of trying to find out what was causing her pain, fatigue, and cognitive and digestive difficulties. "It was frustrating," she says now. "Lots of doctors and lots of tests. Some doctors were understanding, while others were insensitive."

The diagnosis brought with it "a sense of relief at finally having a name for my condition. But I was also frustrated because FM is not accepted by many people as a *real* disorder. I was also a bit frightened because I had no idea where this illness would lead me," she says.

Although Melinda does not sleep well, she is reluctant to take more than minimal medication because of her digestive problems. She endures considerable pain, particularly in her arms and legs. Currently, she takes 10 mg of Flexeril at bedtime and rarely anything else.

Melinda says her husband is "understanding, supportive, and somewhat frustrated at not being able to help me to get well." Her mother and siblings "want me to get myself fixed. My grown daughters seem supportive and a little frightened. They were so used to my being strong and active," she says.

Fibromyalgia has caused her to lower her expectations as far as household chores are concerned. "I've learned to live with a little dust and soap film," she says. "Since I still work, my goal for each weekend is to do laundry, shop for groceries, and do at least one other household chore, such as clean the bathrooms or vacuum and dust, but I don't try to do everything every weekend."

"Fibromyalgia hasn't exactly enhanced my marriage," Melinda says. "I know my husband would like to have more intimate encounters, but he doesn't push me. I think he's a little frustrated, but so am I."

Communication is the key to smoothing the marital relationship, she advises. "I feel lucky that my husband and I have always been able to talk about anything freely. If you try to ignore your feelings of anxiety or fear, it will only come out somewhere else, and I can guarantee it will be ugly."

While she is much less active socially than she used to be, Melinda still plans one activity a week. Keeping from overextending herself is one of her biggest problems, she says. "It is very difficult to say no. I've learned that if I don't, I crater, so I'm getting better at saying, 'I would like to do that, but I just don't have the energy to do it.' "

Melinda has been open with her employer and co-workers about her fibromyalgia. Her boss's reaction is ambivalent. "On the one hand he seems to be very concerned and supportive. On the other hand, he is struggling under the weight of his growing workload. He says he wants to give me more work, but is waiting for me to get better. Talk about pressure. . . ." Her co-workers are also supportive, within limits. "No one is interested in any of the details. They want me to say fine when they ask how I am," she notes. She pinpoints one of fibromyalgia's annoying features when she says, "The problem is that I don't look ill. People expect you to look sick when you say you are."

Assessing the pros and cons of telling people at work about having fibromyalgia, Melinda says, "The advantage is that it helps explain my inability to function at my normal level. The disadvantage is that since it's not exactly an accepted illness, there are those who think it's all in my head and that I'm just trying to escape the pressure of the job."

She has been able to turn some of the most demanding and

stressful of her responsibilities over to others. Her boss wants her to take them back. "But not until I'm well. I don't think that will ever happen," Melinda says.

She also reports that her management style has changed drastically. "I used to be very involved with everything that was going on. Now I rarely leave my office. As a result, I feel that I'm letting everyone down. I'm also afraid that I'm losing my technical skills and that someday I won't be any good to anyone."

CHAPTER TEN

Finding Your Balance

IN the experience of most fibromyalgics who have it under control, living well with fibromyalgia means finding the right balance of sleep, exercise, nutrition, and psychological or spiritual well-being. For each of us, this balance is unique to our needs. It is essential that you understand this and that you work with health care professionals who also understand it. They can help you to find your balance, but they cannot do it for you. That is up to you.

If you have the kind of health care relationship you deserve, you will be encouraged to try a variety of approaches, pay careful attention and make notes about the results, and report back to your health care professional to discuss what to try next. You may be able to do much of this experimentation on your own, seeking a physician's involvement only if you think you need prescription medication. However you do it, it is crucial that you *do it*. If you put the principles in this chapter to work, you can expect to feel better than you do now. You may even find that you can feel *well* most of the time.

I want you to notice that I said *most of the time*, not *all* of the time. You may still experience flare-ups at times, but you will most likely be able to identify the cause of any flare-up and often take steps to avoid that particular cause in the future.

In the list of factors that make up your unique balance—sleep, exercise, nutrition, and emotional status—I put sleep first because of its critical role in relief from pain and fatigue, and in emotional well-being. If you are not sleeping well, that is almost surely the problem to work on first, using the information and suggestions found in chapter 2. The rest of this chapter has suggestions for exercise, nutrition, and emotional status. It will give you ideas about how to monitor and interpret your results and some guidelines for experimenting safely and carefully.

Exercise

Two kinds of exercise help people with fibromyalgia: stretching and aerobic exercise. Here you will find information to help you get started with a daily exercise routine.

Start with stretching. I have found it easier to get out of bed in the morning, an action that most people with fibromyalgia find difficult and painful, if I stretch lying flat on my back first. Yawning or taking a full, deep breath first moves oxygen to the muscles and makes the stretch seem even more effective. Next I sit on the side of my bed and bend forward, my head and arms hanging down and my muscles as relaxed as I can get them to be. I don't push, but simply let the weight of my head pull on my spine. This simple stretching has become habit for me; on the rare occasions that I forget, I know it as soon as I stand up.

There is much more to stretching than this, of course. You can find books and videotapes on stretching listed in Appendix A. If you breathe well and deeply while you stretch, you will increase the benefits. People who have FM often breathe shallowly and don't get enough oxygen to their muscles and brain. Remembering to breathe deeply while stretching won't solve the problem, but it will help significantly.[15]

Gentle daily aerobic exercise is another ingredient in a bodywork regimen that helps many people with fibromyalgia. Aerobic exercise stimulates the production of endorphins, chemical substances that promote the production of serotonin and relieve pain. By increasing serotonin with exercise, and possibly by using medication to prevent it from being reabsorbed prematurely so that it can do its job, you can maximize your chance of getting a good night's sleep.

Aerobic exercise is any activity that gets your heart moving at a rapid rate. To find your target heart rate, subtract your age from 220 and multiply it by 60 percent. This tells you how many heartbeats in a minute will bring you the benefit you seek. When you are exercising, you can check your aerobic rate by taking your pulse for ten seconds. Your ten-second pulse rate should be one-sixth of the one-minute rate. As you increase your aerobic fitness, you may want to work up to 80 percent of 220 minus your age.

This aerobic level of exercise is a goal not a commandment. Many people who have fibromyalgia become discouraged when a doctor suggests that they should exercise. "I hurt too much to move," they say, "and I'll never be able to get my heart going that fast without having a heart attack." You should discuss an exercise program with your personal doctor, nurse practitioner, or health practitioner. For fibromyalgics, some exercise every day is a must.

If you have not been exercising, start small. Walk for a minute the first day if you haven't been walking at all. Walk for two minutes the next day and increase by a minute a day, if that's the best you can do, until you can walk for twenty to thirty minutes. Distance is not important; the goal is to get your heart working aerobically for at least twenty minutes every day. The best news is that you will feel an improvement long before you reach twenty minutes of aerobic exercise.

Before you begin to exercise, take a moment to stretch and warm up your muscles. Shrug your shoulders in a circular motion, first in one direction, then in the other. Raise one arm over your head and bend toward the opposite side. Raise the other arm and repeat. Stand about one pace away from a wall. Put your hands on the wall at shoulder height. With your feet flat on the floor, bend your elbows and let your straight body lean into the wall, as though you were doing push-ups while standing. Repeat once or twice. Then, in the same position, put one foot ahead of the other, keep both feet flat on the floor, and lean into the wall again, once or twice. Switch the feet and do it again.

Walking is not the only way to exercise—it's just the least expensive. People who have fibromyalgia often have trouble climbing, so if you live in a hilly area you may want to invest in a treadmill. Just be sure that it can be adjusted to be level with the floor. Riding a stationary bike is another good form of exercise. The wheel tension should be light at the start; you can add resistance as time goes by if your knees and leg muscles will put up with it. And if you can't use your legs to exercise, use your arms. There are over-the-door pulley arrangements for people who can only exercise their arms. You can also use two small unopened soup or juice cans as hand weights and get those arms moving. One of the resources listed in the Appendix sells a videotape of exercises for people who cannot stand while they exercise.

Swimming or working out in a pool is an excellent form of exercise for people with fibromyalgia. Exercising in water reduces the effects of gravity, so you do not have to bear as much of your weight while you work out. Water offers all the resistance you need. There are, however, two things to watch out for if you're swimming. Some people are bothered by chlorine and, although disinfectants are necessary to good pool hygiene, many pool managers seem to think that if some chlorine is good, more is better. If the amount of chlorination makes you uncomfortable, speak to the manager or find a better pool. Second, although I have heard from a few people with FM that they feel invigorated after swimming in cool water, most need a pool temperature of between 86° and 92°F. (30° to 33.3° C) and few pools are heated to that degree. Some motels do have heated pools, however, and may allow nonguests to swim for a fee. Some YMCAs have special swim sessions for people who need extra warmth.

If you swim, try to vary your stroke with each lap so that you don't overexercise any one muscle group. But you don't need to know how to swim to get benefit from water exercise. Here are some other things you can do.

- Use a float board under your chest and kick your legs for propulsion. Or hold on to the side of the pool and kick gently.
- "Bicycle" in the water, lying on your back. Move your hands to keep yourself balanced, and move your legs as though you were biking.

- Water-walk. Wear a buoyancy belt or water-ski belt and walk back and forth in the pool.
- Do jumping jacks in the water.

If walking is your exercise of choice, it's a good idea to have an alternative for bad-weather days. Twenty minutes of aerobic exercise three or four days a week is sufficient for people who don't have FM, but the daily repetition of your exercise program is important, for this reason: If exercise is a new discipline for you, it is easiest to keep it up if you leave no room for excuses. Raining outside? Go to the nearest shopping mall and walk—no fair stopping to window shop—for your allotted number of minutes. If you don't walk today, it will be that much easier to skip it tomorrow. You may get away with skipping one exercise session now and then, but if you skip two days in a row, you'll know it when you're trying to sleep.

Another technique that helps to make exercise a part of your life is to set aside a specific time in your day for working out.[16] It is generally understood that you will get the maximum serotonin benefit four or five hours after you exercise, so mid- to late-afternoon aerobics, four to five hours before bedtime, may be best for you. But if you have things you must do then—preparing dinner, or traveling home from work, for example—pick another time, not less than four hours before you normally go to bed.

I have animals to tend first thing in the morning. When I get up, I dress in my sweats, feed and water my sheep and chickens, and get on my stationary bike for half an hour. Then I dress for the day and have breakfast. These activities follow each other as night follows day. If I deviate, the entire day seems out of kilter. This may sound compulsive, but it is also practical. Having scheduled it so, I never have to make a new decision about whether to exercise. I make one exception to the daily routine: I do not exercise on Sunday. I give myself one day off a week because I can get away with it; my sleep does not suffer on Sunday night, as long as I get to bed at my regular time. Taking one day off removes the feeling of drudgery, and I actually look forward to my Monday morning exercise session.

Some people who have fibromyalgia prefer more formal exercise disciplines such as tai chi and yoga. There are videotapes that can help you learn about them, but a class with a gentle and patient teacher is best. Before you try a class, however, it's advisable to have a private conversation with the teacher. Bring some information about FM, explain your limitations, and satisfy yourself that the teacher will not single you out in class or try to push you beyond what you know to be your limit.

Nutrition

Men have different nutritional needs from women. People who are inactive most of the time have different nutritional needs from athletes. Adults have different nutritional needs from children, and old people's needs are different from both. Smokers and dieters have special needs. Your needs when you are traveling are different from those when you are at home. People recovering from illness or injury have special nutritional needs.

It stands to reason that a multiple-vitamin pill, offering the same formulation to everyone regardless of age, gender, living habits, or health status, is not a satisfactory solution. To find your balance, therefore, explore your unique needs for supplementary vitamins and minerals.

Your library or bookstore can provide many good books on what vitamins and minerals do for our bodies (you will find some suggestions in Appendix A). In the paragraphs that follow, you will find a summary of which vitamins do what for you, and the range of potencies.

Fat-soluble vitamins. These require some fat in order to be absorbed by your body. They can build up to toxic levels, although you'd really have to take several times the dosages mentioned here to make that happen. Fat-soluble vitamins are measured in international units (IU).

Vitamin A: for skin, hair, nails, bones, vision. It aids in the absorption of vitamin D; 10,000 IU is enough for most people.

Beta carotene turns into vitamin A in your body; 15 mg of beta carotene equals 25,000 IU of vitamin A. I would never take that much vitamin A for more than five days, but I take that much beta carotene daily. A deficiency in vitamin A can cause a deficiency in vitamin C.

Vitamin D: for hair, nails, bones, vision. It aids in the absorption of vitamin A; 4,000 IU is enough. The best ratio of A to D is 2.5 to 1. A and D are the vitamins in cod liver oil. You can get A and D capsules combined, which is the easiest way to do it.

Vitamin E: for circulation, stamina. A deficiency can cause leg cramps. Vitamin E is an antioxidant, which some people think is good for preventing cancer; take 400 to 800 IU.

Water-soluble vitamins. Measured in milligrams (mg); 1,000 mg = 1 gram. If you take more than you need, the excess is excreted by your kidneys. You are unlikely to do yourself harm, but you will have very expensive urine.

B complex: for nerves, mental health, the ability to handle stress, and to metabolize food efficiently. A combination of vitamins, they are a complex because they work together; don't take one without taking the rest, or you'll create your own vitamin deficiency. The best way to get the B's is to buy a B-complex tablet or capsule that has 50 or 100 mg of B_6. It will be formulated to have the right proportion of the rest of them. One of these a day is probably enough. One note: If you do this and find your face burning hot for a half hour or so about an hour after you take the first one, this is a reaction to vitamin B_3 (niacin). Do not be alarmed; the reaction is not harmful. You will not get this reaction if you use a B-complex tablet that contains a form of B_3 called niacinamide instead of niacin, and the effect of both is the same. The B-complex vitamins also aid in synthesizing serotonin from the food you eat, which makes it an important nutrient for people with fibromyalgia.

Vitamin C: antiviral, strengthens your immune system, promotes healing, helps overcome stress. Poor appetite is a sure sign of lack of vitamin C; if you take too much you may get ravenously hungry. You may also get diarrhea, but it stops immediately if you cut back. When I feel a cold coming on I take 6 to 8 grams of vitamin C, 2 grams per meal and 2 grams at bedtime, for a few days. The last time I had a cold was 1985. At that time I had run out of vitamins, moved to a new part of the country where I had no immunity to the local viruses, and was also overworked, burned out, and run-down; 500 mg per day is a good normal dose. If you do load up on C to fight off a cold, taper off when you don't need so much anymore; don't just stop cold turkey.

Two minerals that you should consider taking are magnesium and calcium. Magnesium is necessary to metabolize calcium and vitamin C and is essential for nerve and muscle functioning. People who have muscle twitches or cramps may be deficient in magnesium. It is also important in converting blood sugar into energy, for coping with stress, and can aid in fighting depression. Researchers have reported finding low levels of magnesium in the red blood cells of people with fibromyalgia but not in the blood plasma, so it takes a magnesium loading test to discover it. Magnesium may cause diarrhea, so it is usually taken together with calcium, which tends to be constipating. The proper ratio of calcium to magnesium is 2 to 1.

Research into the relationship between amino acids and FM is relatively new, but there are some indications that people with fibromyalgia are deficient in some of the essential amino acids, the building blocks of protein that come to us through our food. This may be related to the fibromyalgic's malabsorption of nutrients in general. Some people with fibromyalgia are reporting good results from taking amino acid supplements, particularly lysine and arginine, which are said to increase levels of human growth hormone. These people say that 500 mg of each is the proper dose, and that the two should always be taken together to avoid creating an imbalance. Reported benefits include better sleep and less pain. I have not tried this myself and cannot recommend it, but it is the kind of thing that I would experiment with if I were not satisfied with my own regimen.

Research has shown that people with fibromyalgia are deficient in the amino acid tryptophan. Tryptophan is present in food, but it is no longer available in the United States as a supplement. Turkey and bananas are two foods particularly rich in tryptophan.

No vitamin, mineral, and amino acid supplement regimen is a substitute for good nutrition. Be sure you eat foods that have:

• as few refined carbohydrates (sugar, white flour, and alcohol) as possible—none at all if you can manage it. Refined sugars rob the system of the B-complex vitamins and trigger an undesirable adrenaline response in many people with fibromyalgia.

• plenty of complex carbohydrates (whole grains especially), vegetables, and fruits, with lots of fiber to keep your digestive system working well and reduce cholesterol in your blood.

• enough protein, whether from meat or nonmeat sources, to provide amino acids needed for muscle growth and repair.

When I was a little girl I had a teacher who liked to say, "You are what you eat." I thought that was really funny then; I don't now. The food that you eat turns into the chemicals that make up your body. There is nothing that you can do for yourself that is more important than giving your body the right food.

Maintaining Good Emotional Health

Your mental state has a profound effect on your fibromyalgia. Your physical pain is real enough, but what goes on in your head can make it more or less bearable.

Take anger, for example. When you are angry, your body reacts: Your adrenaline starts pumping, your heart races, you feel a surge of energy as your blood sugar level soars.

If you have FM, you will probably pay later for this adrenaline surge with overwhelming fatigue, or pain, or both, which is why I address anger first. If you fly off the handle frequently or if you are carrying around a load of anger over your situation or over something that happened at a previous time in your life, you need to work on taking control over your anger. Learn to save it for the few really appropriate times.

Much of this work involves thinking about what *really* requires an angry response. Faced with a potentially anger-producing stimulus, before you do or say anything take one or two really deep breaths. The trick to deep breathing is to try to draw breath into the space about an inch below your navel. If you're doing this right, one breath is enough. Two is for novices. Get good at this. It really helps dissipate anger. If you practice, you will soon learn to run the anger stimulus against your values and needs and you will eventually react appropriately to the situation automatically.

The long-term effect of stress is another example of the interaction of body and mind. The important lesson for people who have fibromyalgia is that stress causes pain and, of course, pain causes stress, so we have to find a way to break the cycle. Stress reduction is an important component of your overall fibromyalgia regimen. Attend a stress management course or workshop if you can. If your health care provider recommends that you learn stress-reduction techniques, don't take it as a suggestion that your pain is of psychological origin. The ability to manage stress will be one more tool in your arsenal to fight fibromyalgia.

Here are some other suggestions for finding your mental and spiritual balance:

• Stop fighting your pain. As long as you fight it, your pain controls you. Physically fighting pain only makes it worse. Concentrate on relaxing the area that hurts, let the pain flow through you, and you will feel it diminish.

• Close your eyes and visualize the place that hurts. Mentally send the area your love and sympathy, give it a hug, and let it rest.

• Distract yourself. Imagine being in a place where there is no pain. Listen to soft, relaxing music and trust it to help you to heal.

• Investigate your pain. Explore what makes it flare up, and try to avoid those situations. Explore what makes it feel better, and make those things happen as often as you can.

• Learn to meditate. Practice mindfulness, the technique of being fully aware of the moment you are in, not the past or the future. Learn to recognize when your stress level increases and what makes it increase.

• Fill your life with people who are kind to you. You may have to deal with some who are unkind, but you can do so on a superficial level. You are not required to keep in your life anyone who is toxic to you. In other words, don't let them get to you.

• Find people who understand what fibromyalgia is like. Join a support group that has a positive outlook. Feelings of loneliness and negativity are the enemies to your balance.

Above all, learn to ask for what you need and to receive it gracefully. One of the great gifts fibromyalgia has given me is the lesson that it is often better to receive than to give. If you think about this stricture that our culture has put on us, that nobody should ever ask for help, you can see how ridiculous it really is. If nobody ever asked for help, then no one would ever have the opportunity to be helpful. I've learned to make my request and to say simply thank you when my request is fulfilled. I try to be helpful in ways that are possible for me, thereby returning my debt to those around me, but I have learned to swallow my pride and admit that I am nothing more than human. Sometimes I can give, sometimes I need to be given to. It's a warm feeling to be human. Let it come.

Listening to Your Body

You are the expert on your own body. Nobody knows it the way you do. But if you are like most people in our society, you have lost the intimate relationship with your body that you had when you were small. If you have had FM since childhood, you learned long ago that you had to ignore pain and fatigue if you were going to accomplish anything. Even if you grew up without fibromyalgia, you had to learn to ignore your own wish to be active, in order to sit in class all day. You may have learned to ignore feeling ill when it was inconvenient for you or those around you to have you sick. You learned to eat when it was time to eat, instead of when you were hungry, and perhaps you were taught to eat everything on your plate whether you liked it or not, whether you were hungry or not. In these and other subtle ways, most of us were taught to ignore our bodies instead of listen to them.

At one time in my life, I put so much energy into ignoring pain that I nearly died. At another time I ignored pain in my lower back until it turned into a full-blown case of sciatica and I could no longer walk. I didn't know any better, but now I know there are times when pain has an important message for us, and we must listen.

But there is another kind of listening to your body that is just as important. It involves paying attention to the effects on your body of everything that happens to it: what you eat, what you breathe in, how you move, how you feel, what you say and hear, what you do, and what is done to you.

If listening to your body becomes a habit, you will know almost immediately whether something is good or bad for you. If you listen to your body, you will take control over your body, and that control is the vital ingredient in living with fibromyalgia. In the next section I suggest some techniques for listening to your body when it tells you about its problems so that you can work on finding solutions.

Troubleshooting Fibromyalgia

You have come to a place where you are ready to start troubleshooting your own version of fibromyalgia. When I started this process for my own case, my approach was much like that of a mechanic troubleshooting an automobile problem or a computer user trying to figure out how to make a particular piece of software work properly. Fortunately, you don't have to be an expert to improve your life with fibromyalgia. Troubleshooting is a step-by-step logical process that anyone can do. These are the steps to follow.

• List the problems to be solved, ranking them from most to least important in terms of the quality of your life.

• List the symptoms of each problem, again ranking them from most to least distressing.

• List all the possible causes for each symptom that you can think of, ranking them from most to least likely in your opinion.

• List all the possible remedies for each symptom, ranking them from most to least desirable in terms of potential side effects, estimated effectiveness, cost, and any other factors that are important to you.

• Choose a problem and symptom and try the remedy that makes the most sense to you, moving through the list of remedies, if necessary, until you find one that works satisfactorily.

• Pay careful attention to your results. Make notes and write up your conclusions so that you don't forget what you did and what happened.

If you are oriented more toward pictures than words, you may prefer to make drawings or diagrams, rather than lists. If you learn better from what you hear than from what you read, you may prefer recording your findings on a tape recorder, rather than writing them down. Whatever method you use to figure out what you need to do to help yourself, the technique remains the same: set priorities, experiment with solutions, and record your results.

If you have a doctor who is well informed about fibromyalgia and willing to support you in your effort to improve your condition, involve your doctor in this troubleshooting approach. This kind of physician can be a valuable resource, a consultant who helps you to figure things out and provides information that you would be otherwise hard pressed to obtain. Some of the chemical approaches you want to try may require a doctor's prescription. Others, such as massage, physical therapy, or classes in stress reduction, may be affordable only if the doctor prescribes them and insurance pays for them. If you have the kind of doctor who will not support your efforts, you may want to make finding the right doctor your first priority.

An important resource that you should not overlook is your pharmacist. Find one who has the patience and interest in you to help you investigate drug interactions, whether the drugs are prescribed by a doctor or purchased off the shelf. The more different substances you take, the greater are the chances for two or more of them to interact in undesirable ways. A good pharmacist is your best line of defense against untoward interactions, and since it's easier to change pharmacists than it is to change doctors—you just go to another drugstore—finding a pharmacist you like and trust is a relatively easy first step in your troubleshooting program.

List the problems to be solved.   Here are some of the fibromyalgia-related problems that you may want to list: sleep, musculoskeletal pain, visceral/organ pain, irritable bowel, urethral syndrome, headache/migraine, fatigue, menstrual problems, emotional problems, circulatory problems. List them in order of their importance to the quality of your life.

List the symptoms of each problem.   Under sleep, for example, you might list that you have trouble falling asleep, that you have trouble staying asleep, that you wake up at 3:00 A.M. and cannot get back to sleep, a combination of these, or something different. Do this for each of the problems on your list, and arrange them according to their importance in the quality of your life.

List the possible causes for each symptom. To continue the sleep example, think about what keeps you from falling asleep: worries? street noise? pain? someone snoring? sleep apnea? Try to relax when you think about possible causes. Let your mind focus on thinking about what happens (or does not happen) before these symptoms appear. This may take some time, but don't give it more than forty-eight hours or you may never get back to this project. You can always add things later. In fact, as you continue this process, you may want to spend some time reading articles in magazines or medical journals about the symptoms you feel you know least about. When you feel you have enough to work with, or within two days at most, arrange these possibilities according to their importance in causing the symptom.

List the possible remedies for each symptom. Some symptoms will lead you back to another of the problems to be solved, which is why you may like the idea of drawing a diagram. Don't worry about this. You'll get to that problem before long, and you may want to change your priorities at that point. Others are simpler: Is somebody's snoring keeping you awake? Possible remedies include an antisnoring device for the snorer, earplugs for you, separate bedrooms, and whatever you can think of. Take another forty-eight hours if you need to, but don't let this step be your last in this project. Remember to consider all kinds of possibilities that make sense to you, some of which may be medicinal, nutritional, herbal, physical—massage, for example—and more. When you have enough possible remedies to get started, arrange them in order of your estimate of the likelihood that they may help and are feasible.

Try one thing at a time. Pick your number one problem, one or more of its symptoms, and, ordinarily, one of the possible remedies. Pick more than one symptom at a time to address, or more than one possible remedy, only if they are related and you can't see how to do one without the other. For example, you might choose to address street noise and snoring simultaneously, by using earplugs and getting your sleepmate to try an antisnore device. You should not, however, try to address sleep and pain at the same time. I had to make this choice. I gambled that my pain was not severe enough to keep me awake, if only I could get to real, restful sleep. As it turned out, once I solved my sleep problem my pain was almost gone. Your experience may be completely opposite, but you'll probably be more successful if you pick one to work on first.

Listen to your body.   Keep careful notes. Describe the problem, what symptoms you are attacking and how you are attacking them, and record dates and dosages. Note your results in detail: how you felt before you tried it, what happened after you tried it. Do this day by day; most remedies do not work immediately but need time to be effective. Be patient. It may help to set a time limit in advance for each thing you try. For example, if you try earplugs and an antisnore device because you think your sleeping partner's snoring is the major cause of your insomnia, it could take two or three days to know whether you've found a solution. It may take that long to get used to the earplugs and to get your mind geared to anticipate sleep rather than wakefulness, but it shouldn't take more than a week. Medicines, nutritional supplements, or herbs might take days, weeks, or months to take effect. If you know enough to try a nonmedicinal remedy, or your doctor knows enough to prescribe a drug, then you should be able to estimate how much time you give the trial before moving on to something else. Of course, with few exceptions, if something you try soon makes you feel worse, you should probably stop it and reconsider.

It is impossible to overestimate the importance of keeping records. A week from now, maybe sooner, you will forget what you did and how you felt today. Decisons are much harder to make if you have incomplete information about what you have tried and what the results were. I suggest that you use left-hand pages in a notebook to record what you did, and right-hand pages to record the results.

CASE HISTORY: CANDY, 44, FORMER BANK MANAGER

Candy was thirty-two when she first became ill with "a rash from head to toe and a fever of 101°." Her regular internist, Dr. A., was on vacation. The doctor who was covering for Dr. A. referred Candy to a dermatologist in the same medical facility. The dermatologist said Candy had either measles, which she had had as a child, or a virus. In either case, he said, it would go away within a week or so.

The rash went away, just as the dermatologist had said, but it was replaced by a rash on Candy's face, accompanied by an overwhelming fatigue. Over the next year, she developed pain in her neck, shoulders, arms, hands, fingers, hips, knees, feet, and toes. Dr. A sent her to a rheumatologist, who ordered a long series of tests that revealed nothing. As the pain and fatigue increased, Dr. A. tried a succession of NSAIDs, but nothing helped. "Finally, out of desperation on both our parts, he put me on prednisone, a steroid," Candy says. "It was a miracle. I felt like me again. Very little pain, and no more fatigue." The steroid allowed Candy to continue in her role as "a full-time supermom, bank branch manager, and homemaker, with lots of stress." For the next two years, the prednisone worked well. During this time, Dr. A. retired. His successor was Dr. B., a young internist.

Suddenly Candy, then thirty-four, began having irregular heartbeats and panic attacks. "I had been warned that prednisone shouldn't be taken for a long time. I was sure the prednisone was the cause of the irregular heartbeat," she says. Dr. B. sent her to another doctor for evaluation. "This doctor yelled at me, saying there was nothing wrong with me and that if I just lost some weight and was more physically active, I would be fine. I was in tears when I left," Candy recalls.

She went back to Dr. B., who suggested that she see a psychiatrist. "I knew I didn't need that, and I also knew that Dr. B.

was not for me. I stopped the prednisone and decided I would take care of myself," she says.

Candy recalls the next few years as "a terror: more pain and more fatigue." She developed irritable bowel syndrome (IBS), swollen glands, and migraine headaches. "I was having problems remembering and thinking. I could no longer work," she says. Without her income, she and her husband were forced to sell their house and move in with Candy's parents. "Luckily, we had their support," says Candy. After having lived with her parents for a year, she developed the all-over rash once again. Her mother insisted that she consult a doctor.

Candy went to Dr. C., an internist associated with her mother's doctor. He examined her, ran some tests that revealed nothing, and sent her to Dr. D. at a major university hospital, saying, "If Dr. D. can't tell you what is wrong, then nobody can.' I figured that if Dr. C. believed there was something wrong with me, then I was willing to see the doctor that he recommended, but I did so very reluctantly."

She had to wait a month to see Dr. D. "By the time I finally had my appointment, I was a real mess. Everything hurt. I could hardly think." Her visit to Dr. D. was the first time she heard the term *fibromyalgia*. "I was shocked! I had a syndrome! It had a name! I really wasn't crazy!" Candy says. Dr. D. prescribed Elavil (amitriptyline) "to treat a sleep disorder I didn't even realize I had." He sent Candy back to Dr. C. with suggestions for treating her fibromyalgia.

Dr. C. is a firm believer in the team approach to treating FM, so Candy had a variety of therapeutic treatments in the year that followed her diagnosis, but showed very little progress. Dr. C. told her he considered her fully disabled, and Candy applied for Social Security disability. Also, under Dr. C.'s guidance, she took biofeedback training to learn deep-relaxation techniques. She also took a course in pain management. "It wasn't until I took the pain management course that I really faced the fact that I am disabled and confronted my losses due to FM. Until then, I had always had it in the back of my mind that I would be well enough someday to go back to my old job. Now I realized that this would probably not happen, that at best I may be able to work part time, sometime in the future," she says. "I've lost a lot: my health, my fast-track job, my home, my mobility, lots of friends, and a social life, all due to FM."

Candy sees anger and denial as her "real enemies. I have learned to face my losses, grieve for them, and move on. It's a long process and I'm still struggling," she adds.

Despite all her losses, Candy believes that she has gained more than she has lost. "Living with a chronic illness isn't easy, but it compels you to appreciate the little things in life and strive for inner peace," she says. "Illness has a way of showing you what is really important. It frees you to look inside yourself, to see what a strong person you can become. By writing in a daily journal, meditation, and with the help of a wonderful support group, I have learned that I'm not alone. There are millions of people just like me. With the support of real friends, a loving family, and by the grace of God, I will survive."

Epilogue

FIBROMYALGIA is, for the most part, invisible. Most of us look much younger, and far healthier, than we feel. We probably look this way because the tightness of our facial muscles keeps them from sagging with age. I once saw a woman with FM wearing a button that said, "I look better than I feel."

I believe that you don't feel well. I also believe that you are going to feel much better shortly after you find your own balance. Several studies have shown that people with fibromyalgia do indeed start feeling better when they start taking control over their condition. Read these words from one paper, published in 1995, in which the investigator asked a group of women with FM to describe how they live with it. "The women described living with FM as struggling to maintain balance. This involves recalling perceived normality, searching for a diagnosis, finding out, and moving on [that is], transcending the illness. . . . Over time the illness moves from being a primary life focus to being part of the backdrop of the lives of women with FM."

You can do at least that well, and I think you can do even better. Read this message, from a woman who loves horses and riding. I had met her a year earlier, at a time when she felt she had lost everything. Let her inspire you.

> Today I got my life back! I drove past fields of hay. I have flies in my camper and my boots have shavings in the seams. I smell like a horse and I'm soaking wet and my dog loves me. I've made arrangements to ride two or three times a week on the

same horse, and my saddle now proudly sits in the tack room. I rode in the arena, outside in the ring, through a field and down the driveway. I even trotted (although very badly). I'm going to have to do this on loan money but I'm investing in my future and I believe in me. When I ride, I push myself past the pain and exhaustion because I've trained myself to do this for so many years. I feel that I've turned a corner physically and will be able to do this whenever I wish. To my doctors and others who said I would never ride again, I say a heartfelt NEIGHHHHHHHHHHHH!

I've had FM almost all my life. For the most part, my good days have outnumbered my bad days, although some of the bad days were terrible. If you are in a bad place now, I want you to believe that good times will come again. The challenge is to figure out what works for you, and then stick with it. Please believe me. A positive mental attitude is a powerful tool with which to work. You *can* figure out this puzzle, and you *can* live well again. Be patient and determined, and you will prevail.

Resources

EXERCISE

"Fibromyalgia Exercise Video": Stretching, prepared by two of the foremost fibromyalgia experts, Robert M. Bennett, M.D., and Sharon R. Clark, Ph.D.

>National Fibromyalgia Research Association
>P.O. Box 500
>Salem, OR 97308
>503-588-1411

"Thera-Fit While You Sit," a complete upper-body aerobic workout for people who cannot stand while exercising.

>The Hygienic Corporation
>1245 Home Avenue
>Akron, OH 44310
>216-633-8460
>Fax: 216-633-9359

>The Hygienic Corporation of Canada
>14 Northrup Crescent
>St. Catherines, ON L2M 7N7
>800-461-0574
>905-937-5957

Exercise information for people who can't exercise standing up is also available from:

Seat-A-Robics Inc.
P.O. Box 630064
Little Neck, NY 11363-0064
718-631-4007

The "ROM Dance," a video of exercises to improve range of motion.

The ROM Institute
3601 Memorial Drive
Madison, WI 53704
608-249-6670
Fax: 608-249-7466

Anderson, Bob. *Stretching*. Bolinas, California: Shelter Publications, 1980.
Illustrations show right and wrong ways to stretch.

FIBROMYALGIA

Backstrom, Gayle. *When Muscle Pain Won't Go Away*. Dallas: Taylor Publishing Co., 1995.
Appendix lists organizational resources and professionals.

MYOFASCIAL PAIN SYNDROME

Cummings, Sally A. *Trigger Points: Understanding Myofascial Pain and Discomfort*. Skokie, IL: Anatomical Chart Co., 1994.
Diagrams and charts of trigger points and exercises to relieve them.

Simons, David G., M.D. *Myofascial Pain Syndrome Due to Trigger Points*. Monograph, available free from Gebauer Company, 9410 St. Catherine Avenue, Cleveland, OH 44104; 800-321-9348.

Starlanyl, Devin and Mary Ellen Copeland. *Fibromyalgia and Chronic Myofascial Pain Syndrome: A Survival Manual*. Oakland, CA: New Harbinger, Spring 1996.
Focus is on myofascial pain and trigger points.

Travell, Janet and David Simons. *Myofascial Pain and Dysfunction: The Trigger Point Manual*. Baltimore: Williams & Wilkins, 1983.

Travell, Janet and David Simons. *Myofascial Pain and Dysfunction: The Trigger Point Manual, vol. II*. Baltimore: Williams & Wilkins, 1992.

The two-volume classic work on myofascial pain. Very technical; a medical textbook. Volume I covers the upper body, volume II the lower body.

NUTRITION

Mindell, Earl. *Earl Mindell's Vitamin Bible.* New York: Warner Books, 1991. Detailed information on vitamins, minerals, and other nutritional supplements.

PAIN AND STRESS MANAGEMENT

Kabat-Zinn, Jon. *Full Catastrophe Living: Using the Wisdom of Your Body and Mind to Face Stress, Pain, and Illness.* New York: Dell Publishing, 1990.

McKenzie, Robin. *Treat Your Own Back.* Minneapolis: Orthopedic Physical Therapy, 1985 (phone 800-367-7393).
————. *Treat Your Own Neck.* Minneapolis: Orthopedic Physical Therapy, 1983.
Two books with easy-to-follow instructions for relief of back and neck pain.

SELF-HELP

McCall, Timothy B., M.D., *Examining Your Doctor: A Patient's Guide to Avoiding Harmful Medical Care.* New York: Birch Lane Press, 1995.
Inside information on how to manage your relationship with your physician.

Pollin, Irene. *Taking Charge: Overcoming the Challenges of Long-Term Illness.* New York: Random House, 1994.
Advice for people learning to live with chronic illness.

PRODUCTS

Hand-Eze gloves provide warmth, support, and massage for hands engaged in typing, needlework, etc. Sold in mail-order catalogs and at sewing supply stores, or call:

Dome, Inc.
800-432-4352

For dry mouth caused by medication:

Oral Balance saliva substitute
800-922-5856

Moist Plus saliva supplement
800-234-1464

Adaptive and assistive devices:

Fred Sammons, Inc.
P.O. Box 32
Brookfield, IL 60513-0032
800-323-5547
708-325-1700

House of Canes & Walking Sticks
800-451-0745

AdaptAbility
800-937-3482
TTY: 800-688-4889

Allergy-free products:

Allergy Alternative
440 Godfrey Drive
Windsor, CA 95492
800-838-1514

Back and neck rolls:

Orthopedic Physical Therapy Products
800-367-7393

Vitamins, minerals, nutritional supplements:

Ecological Formulas	800-888-4585
Hickey Chemists	800-724-5566
KAL Supplements	800-755-4525
L&H Vitamins	800-221-1152
Life Services Supplements	800-542-3230
Canada	800-345-9105

Nutrition Plus	800-241-9236
Peggy's Health Center	800-862-9191
Smart Products	800-858-6520
Vitamin Express	415-564-8160
Vitamin Research Products	800-VRP-24HR
The Vitamin Shop	800-223-1216

Sources of tryptophan and 5-htp

L-tryptophan sources:

Ronald Sturtz
BIOS Biochemicals
8987-309 E. Tanque Verde #340
Tucson, AZ 85749
520-749-8724

Chem-Lab Supplies
1060 Ortega Way, Unit C
Placentia, CA 92670
714-630-7902

Sources of 5-htp: by prescription:

Medical Center Pharmacy
10721 Main Street
Fairfax, VA 22030
800-723-7455
Fax: 703-591-3604

College Pharmacy
833 N. Tejon Street
Colorado Springs, CO 80903
800-888-9358
719-634-4861

Source of 5-htp, no prescription required:

Cosmic Sales and Marketing
800-359-9896

Life Link
445 Lierly Lane
Arroyo Grande, CA 93420
805-473-1389

ORGANIZATIONS AND INFORMATION SOURCES

American Association of Disabled Persons
800-642-8775

Americans with Disabilities Act hotline
800-466-4232
800-949-4232
Direct connection to local ADA office.

Guaifenesin Treatment Information
R. Paul St. Amand, M.D.
4560 Admiralty Way, Suite 355
Marina Del Rey, CA 90292
310-577-7510

Job Accommodations Network
800-232-9675

National Chronic Pain Outreach Association (NCPOA)
7979 Old Georgetown Road
Bethesda, MD 20814-2429
301-652-4948 or 202-408-9514

National Family Caregivers Association
9223 Longbranch Parkway
Silver Springs, MD 20901
Advice and support for healthy relatives of disabled people.

National Organization of Social Security Claims Representatives
800-431-2804
Provides lists of lawyers with expertise in Social Security disability.

Restless Legs Syndrome Foundation
1904 Banbury Road
Raleigh, NC 27608

Sexual Information and Education Council of the U.S. (SIECUS)
32 Washington Place
New York, NY 10003
212-673-3850
A clearinghouse for information and services relating to sex information. Provides information on sex for disabled individuals.

The TMJ Association
6418 W. Washington Boulevard
Wauwatosa, WI 53213
414-259-3223

Well Spouse Foundation
610 Lexington Avenue, Suite 813
New York, NY 10022
800-838-0879 (to leave message)
212-644-1241 (live contact/closed Tuesdays)
Gives emotional support to spouses of the chronically ill; produces a
bimonthly newsletter.

FIBROMYALGIA ORGANIZATIONS

Association de la Fibromyosite du Quebec
643 rue Notre Dame
Repentigny, PQ J6A 2W1
Fibromyalgia information in the French language.

FIBROM-L, the Internet fibromyalgia discussion group provides information and support for people with fibromyalgia and their family members.
  To subscribe, send electronic mail to listserv@mitvma.mit.edu. For the
message, write subscribe FIBROM-L Your Name. There is no charge
other than what you pay your Internet service provider for online time.
Messages sent to fibrom-l also appear on the newsgroup alt.med.fibromy-
algia.

Fibromyalgia Alliance of America, Inc.
P.O. Box 16600
Washington, DC 20041-6600
202-310-1818
Fax: 703-620-1525

Fibromyalgia Alliance of America
P.O. Box 21990
Columbus, OH 43221-0990
(614) 457-4222

Fibromyalgia Association of Greater Washington (FMAGW)
12210 Fairfax Towne Center, Suite 500
Fairfax, VA 22033
703-790-2324

National Fibromyalgia Research Association
P.O. Box 500
Salem, OR 97308
503-588-1411

NIH/National Arthritis and Musculoskeletal and Skin Diseases
Information Clearinghouse
9000 Rockville Pike
Bethesda, MD 20892
301-495-4484

Ontario Fibromyalgia Association
250 Bloor Street E., Suite 901
Toronto, Ontario, M4W 3P2

PUBLICATIONS

Fibromyalgia Network
P.O. Box 31750
Tucson, AZ 85751-1750
800-853-2929
520-290-5508
Fax: 520-290-5550
Publishes a quarterly newsletter; can provide names of fibromyalgia-aware physicians by geographical area.

Journal of Musculoskeletal Pain, published quarterly by Haworth
    Medical Press
10 Alice Street
Binghamton, NY 13904
800-342-8678
Important, professional-level medical journal devoted to research in fibromyalgia and related conditions.

Tips for Making Your Life Easier

As I gathered material for this book, dozens of people told me about ways they make their life easier. Many have appeared throughout the book; here are some more.

AROUND THE HOUSE

• If your freezer requires defrosting, next time you do it, spray the inside of the freezer and the coils on the back with a nonstick vegetable spray. Next time you defrost, the ice will lift off the freezer in sheets. Great for people who can't let their hands get cold.

• Use paper plates to save dish washing. You can find recyclable paper plates that are sturdy enough for dinner use.

• Collect easy, one-dish recipes. On a day when you need to be still, list the ingredients and quantities required of each on a sticky-backed note. Then, when you plan meals, you'll be a step ahead in preparing your shopping list.

• You don't have to grate cheese. Most hard cheese, such as cheddar, can be wrapped tightly and frozen in usable amounts. When it defrosts, it crumbles in your hand.

• For a quick ice pack, use a bag of frozen peas or corn.

• To save steps when you go food shopping, make a map of the location in your market of items you use, then use that map to make your shopping list. Picture yourself walking up and down the aisles, and write down what you need in each aisle.

• Keep a supply of leftovers and ready-to-eat ingredients in a specific section of the refrigerator where people can help themselves to what they like and heat their own meal.

• Label everything you put in the refrigerator and freezer so that you can send others to get what you need.

• Assemble all the ingredients before you start to cook anything to reduce the possibility of errors, particularly on days when the brain fog is thick. If you put the premeasured ingredients on pieces of waxed paper, you will minimize clean-up chores.

• Serve food from the pot or pan to the plate to minimize clean-up work.

• Do your mixing or pouring over or just beside the sink. If you spill, there's less to clean up.

• Give children old enough to open the refrigerator their own plastic water bottle with a straw built into the lid. Let them be responsible for keeping it filled and replaced in the refrigerator.

• When lifting and carrying, hold things close to your body instead of dangling from your hands.

• Avoid twisting at the waist when you are carrying or holding anything.

• Test the weight of objects by sliding them before lifting them. Anything too heavy to slide easily is too heavy to lift.

• If you must carry things in your hands, distribute the weight evenly on both sides.

• Make a platform about eighteen inches high to elevate the clothes dryer and reduce the amount of lifting and bending involved in getting wet clothes out of the washer and into the dryer.

• In the garden, use knee pads or a kneeler that reverses to be a low seat. Rest for fifteen minutes every hour. Take a water jug with you to the garden; drink often and don't let yourself dehydrate. Do things the lazy way, with levers and rollers for moving heavy things.

• After gardening or any bent-over or heavy work, lie down on the floor on your stomach and concentrate on relaxing your back muscles for about fifteen minutes. You can often avoid back pain this way.

• Use a wheeled cart or table in the kitchen to move ingredients from the refrigerator to the work counter, or to move dishes from the table to the sink. Sit on a high, wheeled stool while you work at the kitchen counter, and at the sink or stove.

AT WORK OR SCHOOL

• If you have material to study or memorize, read it aloud. Many people learn better if they both see and hear the information. You might also tape record what you are reading, and play it for review when you are driving or resting.

• Use a white board and dry marker to list tasks and deadlines; cross them out as you are finished. This will allow you to see progress during the day, and will remind you of what you have done.

• Put writing implements, scissors, and other desk items on a lazy susan on top of your desk to minimize the amount of reaching you must do.

• Be ever mindful of posture and ergonomics; ask for a proper chair, wrist rest, and whatever else you need at your desk to avoid repetitive-strain injury. You should not need to invoke the ADA to get such improvements; they are good for everyone not only for people with fibromyalgia.

WHILE DRIVING OR TRAVELING

• Buy a key ring for your house and car keys that fits over your wrist. When you come home, open the door and slip the key ring over the door knob on the inside of the door. When you go out, slip the ring over your wrist. If you're driving, slip it over your wrist when you turn off the ignition.

• Don't get caught with nothing to drink. Carry a plastic pint bottle of water from home so that you don't have to settle for coffee or a sugar- and caffeine-loaded soft drink.

• Ride the transport cart at the airport; ask a ticket agent to call one for you, if necessary. Don't think you have to be severely handicapped to catch a ride; airline personnel do it all the time.

• On the airplane, put one of those little airline pillows in the small of your back.

• Most people dehydrate on airplanes; the air is drier than that in the Sahara Desert. Ask a flight attendant for a bottle of mineral water or seltzer during beverage service and every hour or two during the flight. Avoid coffee and alcoholic drinks in flight. They make dehydration worse.

• Dress comfortably for travel—loose clothing, flat shoes.

• Within reason, the less you pack the more you will enjoy the trip.

• Pack a carry-on bag with whatever you must have until noon the day after you arrive—medications, toothbrush, a change of underwear at a minimum. Check everything else through to your destination. If your bag gets misdirected, you'll be only mildly inconvenienced. Most lost luggage is returned the next day.

• Time zone changes bother people who have fibromyalgia more than most people. Here is a way to minimize jet lag: Counting the day of your trip as day 5, begin on day 1 to alternate days of low-calorie (about 900), high-complex carbohydrate (fruits and vegetables, mainly) meals and high-calorie (about 2,000), high-protein meals. The day of the trip should be a low-calorie day. On the flight, pass up alcoholic drinks for lots of water. Sparkling water gets into your bloodstream faster than plain water. Mineral water is better than tap water; all airlines carry both kinds of bottled water, but some will give them to you only if you ask. Don't let yourself dehydrate. As soon as possible after arrival, get out into the daylight (sun, if you're lucky) without sunglasses for about three hours. Walk as much of that time as you can. Do the same thing on the way home.

• Consider taking 3 to 6 mg of melatonin when you want to go to sleep at your destination city, or move your internal clock around before you leave home by going to bed an hour earlier or later each night for the number of hours that your destination is ahead or behind your time zone.

• Reserve an aisle or bulkhead seat to give you the flexibility to get up and move around during the flight without climbing over other passengers.

• Exercise while seated to reduce stiffness and swelling. Flex and relax your calf muscles and wiggle your toes.

• If it's important to be at your best soon after you arrive from a long distance, try to fly business or first class. The seats are better and roomier, and there's more room to move about the cabin. If you're vacationing a long way from home, it may be worthwhile to shorten your time away by a day or two and spend that money on upgrading your ticket.

PERSONAL CARE

• To minimize the discomfort of switching from standard to daylight saving time or the reverse, try resetting your internal clock gradually, fifteen minutes at a time, every three days. To go from daylight saving to standard time in the autumn, twelve days before the official change, start taking whatever you use for sleep fifteen minutes earlier than usual. Move your medication time back fifteen minutes every three days, and you'll have to adjust your sleep time by only fifteen minutes the night the clocks are reset. Do the same thing in the spring, only taking your sleep medications fifteen minutes later.

• If you are scheduled for dental work, take extra vitamin C two or three days before your appointment. Before you leave for the dentist's office, take the maximum permissible dose of the NSAID you normally use. Don't wait until you're already in pain to seek pain relief. You will probably need to take much less if you do it this way.

• Ask the dentist not to put adrenaline or epinephrine in the needle with the Novocain. The numbing will wear off sooner and you may need a second injection, but you will avoid the aftereffects that most people with fibromyalgia experience from the adrenaline surge.

• If you find it painful to have blood drawn for laboratory tests, ask the technician to let you rub an ice cube over the area first to numb it.

• If your arms get tired when you blow-dry your hair, attach a plastic tube or wooden rod to extend the handle so that you do not have to raise your arms so high.

• If you have trouble swallowing pills, try this: Take a good long drink of water to lubricate your throat. Hold the pill(s) in your nondominant hand and the drink in your dominant hand. Put your hand with the pills in it against your mouth. Toss the pills back into your throat while tilting your head back about 45 degrees. Aim for your tonsils, not the back of your tongue. Quickly toss the water at your tonsils and swallow a big gulp. Wash it all down with the rest of the water. You don't have to gulp it now. The goal is to get the pills as far back in your throat as possible and immediately wash them down in a flood of water.

• So-called panic attacks are most often caused by an adrenaline surge after eating something containing sugar. A fast way to stop the surge is to drink a glass of milk with at least 2 percent butterfat content. The lactose in the milk brings blood sugar up quickly. The butterfat holds it stable.

Glossary

alpha-delta sleep anomaly • A phenomenon in which alpha (awake) brain waves intrude into delta (deep) sleep.

apnea • A condition in which one stops breathing during sleep, resulting in a sudden awakening. A possible cause of fibromyalgia, it is more common among men and is readily treated.

delta sleep • Slow-wave, deep sleep.

dysfunction • Difficult or abnormal functioning.

electroencephalogram • A record of the brain's electrical activity.

electromyogram • Abbreviated as EMG, a test of nerves and muscles to determine if there is any damage.

fibromyalgia • More properly, the fibromyalgia syndrome—a set of signs and symptoms that, taken together, indicates a specific disorder whose cause and cure are as yet unknown.

fibromyalgic • A person who has fibromyalgia.

HMO • Health maintenance organization, a company that may be organized for profit that provides comprehensive health care to members.

melatonin • A hormone secreted by the pineal gland at night that promotes sleep.

myoclonus • A condition involving muscle jerks, spasms, or contractions; sleep myoclonus—muscle jerks in the limbs before or during sleep—is often part of the fibromyalgia syndrome.

myofascial pain syndrome (MPS) • A condition involving pain in the connective tissue surrounding muscles, thought to be caused by trigger points.

neurotransmitter • A chemical that transmits messages between nerves.

NSAID • Nonsteroidal anti-inflammatory drug; for example aspirin, ibuprofen, and naproxen.

serotonin • A neurotransmitter that affects sleep, appetite, mood, and the perception of pain.

somatotropin • Growth hormone, secreted by the pituitary gland and thought to effect muscle repairs.

syndrome • A collection of signs and symptoms.

tender points • Places on the body that are exquisitely tender to the touch. People with fibromyalgia have tender points in predictable locations.

trigger points • Particularly taut places in the muscles associated with myofascial pain syndrome.

Notes

1. Luff, A. J.: The various forms of fibrositis and their treatment. *British Medical Journal* 1913; 1:756–60.

2. Goldenberg, D.: Fibromyalgia syndrome: An emerging but controversial condition. *JAMA* 1987; 257:2782–87.

3. Bennett, R.: Fibromyalgia. *JAMA* 1987; 257:2802–2803.

4. Granges, G. and G. Littlejohn: Prevalence of myofascial pain syndrome in fibromyalgia syndrome and regional pain syndrome: A comparative study. *Journal of Musculoskeletal Pain* 1993; 1(2):19–35.

5. Simons, D. G.: Myofascial pain syndrome due to trigger points, chapter 45. *Rehabilitation Medicine.* J. Goodgold, ed. C. V. Mosby Co., St. Louis, 1988; 686–723.

6. Yunus, M. B.: Research in fibromyalgia and myofascial pain syndromes: Current status, problems, and future directions. *Journal of Musculoskeletal Pain* 1993; 1(1):23–41.

7. Moldofsky, H. D. et al: Musculoskeletal symptoms and non-REM sleep disturbance in patients with "fibrositis syndrome" and healthy subjects. *Psychosomatic Medicine* 1975; 37:341.

8. van Denderen, J. C.; Boersma, J. W.; Zeinstra, P.; Hollander, A. P.; van Neerbos, B. R.: Physiological effects of exhaustive physical exercise in primary fibromyalgia syndrome (PFS): Is PFS a disorder of neuroendocrine reactivity? Department of Rheumatology, Rijnstate Hospital, Arnhem, The Netherlands. *Scandinavian Journal of Rheumatology* 1992; 21(1):35–7.

9. Buskila, D., Press, J., Gedalia, A., Klein, M., Neumann, L., Boehm, R., Sukenik, S.: Assessment of nonarticular tenderness and prevalence of fibromyalgia in children. *Journal of Rheumatology* 1993 Feb.; 20(2):368–70.

10. Thomas Romano M. D., quoted in the Fibromyalgia Network newsletter, Jan. 92, p 4.

11. Pellgrino, M. and Waylonis, G. et al.: Familial occurrence of primary fibromyalgia. *Arch Phys Med Rehabil,* Jan. 1989.

12. Sigal, L. H., Patella, S. J.: Lyme arthritis as the incorrect diagnosis in pediatric and adolescent fibromyalgia. *Pediatrics* 1992 Oct;90(4):523–8.

13. Michael Goldberg, M.D., a pediatrician, in Fibromyalgia Network newsletter, July 93, p. 13.

14. Gedalia, A., Press, J., Klein, M., Buskila, D.: Joint hypermobility and fibromyalgia in schoolchildren. *Ann Rheum Dis* 1993 Jul;52(7):494–6.

15. Fibromyalgia Network newsletter, July, 92, p. 8. James Daly, M.D., pulmonary specialist at Harbor-UCLA, did exercise-to-exhaustion studies on 34 CFS patients, including 22 who met criteria for FMS.

16. McCain, G. A., et al.: A controlled study of the effects of a supervised cardiovascular fitness training program on manifestations of primary fibromyalgia. *Arthritis Rheum* 31:1135, 1988.

Background and Overview Articles

Ahles, T. A.; Khan, S. A.; Yunus, M. B.; Spiegel, D. A.; Masi, A. T.: Psychiatric status of patients with primary fibromyalgia, patients with rheumatoid arthritis, and subjects without pain: a blind comparison of DSM-III diagnoses. *American Journal of Psychiatry* 1991 Dec; 148(12):1721–26.

Bennett, R. M.; Clark, S. R.; Campbell, S. M.; Burckhardt, C. S.: Low levels of somatomedin C in patients with the fibromyalgia syndrome. A possible link between sleep and muscle pain. *Arthritis Rheum* 1992 Oct;35(10):1113–36.

Goldenberg, D. L.: Fibromyalgia syndrome. An emerging but controversial condition. Review Article: 62 Refs. *JAMA* 1987 May 22–29;257(20): 2782–87.

Hench, P. K.: Evaluation and differential diagnosis of fibromyalgia. Approach to diagnosis and management. Review Article: 17 Refs. *Rheum Dis Clin North Am* 1989 Feb;15(1):19–29.

Henriksson, C. M.: Longterm effects of fibromyalgia on everyday life. A study of 56 patients. *Scandinavian Journal of Rheumatology* 1994;23(1): 36–41.

Jacobsen, S.: Chronic widespread musculoskeletal pain—the fibromyalgia syndrome. Review Article: 361 Refs. *Dan Med Bull* 1994 Nov;41(5): 541–64.

Martinez, J. E.; Ferraz, M. B.; Sato, E. I.; Atra, E.: Fibromyalgia versus rneumatoid arthritis: A longitudinal comparison of the quality of life. *Journal of Rheumatology* 1995 Feb;22(2):270–4.

Moldofsky, H.: Fibromyalgia, sleep disorder and chronic fatigue syndrome. Review Article: 48 Refs. *Ciba Found Symp* 1993;173:262–71; discussion 272–79.

Puttini, P. S.; Caruso I: Primary fibromyalgia syndrome and 5-hydroxy-L-tryptophan: a 90-day open study. *J Int Med Res* 1992 Apr;20(2):182–89.

Rosen, N. B.: Physical medicine and rehabilitation approaches to the management of myofascial pain and fibromyalgia syndromes. 100 References *Baillieres Clinical Rheumatology* 1994 Nov;8(4):881–916.

Schaefer, K. M.: Struggling to maintain balance: a study of women living with fibromyalgia. *J Adv Nurs* 1995 Jan;21(1):95–102.

Waylonis, G. W.; Perkins, R. H.: Post-traumatic fibromyalgia. A long-term follow-up. *Am J Phys Med Rehabil* 1994 Nov–Dec;73(6):403–12.

Wolfe, F.; Aarflot, T.; Bruusgaard, D.; Henriksson, K. G.; et al.: Fibromyalgia and disability. Report of the Moss International Working Group on medico-legal aspects of chronic widespread musculoskeletal pain complaints and fibromyalgia. *Scandinavian Journal of Rheumatology* 1995;24(2):112–18.

Index